I0518158

Praise for *My LimanAde Life*

It was serendipity that brought Joan Liman into my life after she heard me speaking on an old NPR interview about Amas Musical Theatre, a non-profit performing arts organization. Little did I know that this chance encounter would ignite her tireless commitment to Amas Musical Theatre—as a volunteer, board member, and former board president. Joan's roller-coaster journey—from physician to educator to surviving life-threatening illnesses—culminates in the fulfillment of her childhood dreams: Immersion in the world of musical theater. Her memoir, both wickedly funny and bravely honest, reads like a gripping theatrical production. Brace yourself for a thrilling ride and prepare to fall in love with Joan—the way I already have.

~Donna Trinkoff, Artistic Producer, Amas Musical Theatre

Joan and I became friends through our shared involvement with Yiddishkayt Initiative, a not-for-profit organization dedicated to celebrating and promoting Jewish history, life, and culture. We shared a common background as physicians but easily related through the rare quality of having powerful creative talents that we had separately and individually brought to successful careers in parallel with our medical careers. Her title, *My LimanAde Life* is a perfectly descriptive, pun-constructive demonstration of her humor and wit, while summing up the theme of her book. Her story is both funny and uplifting, sprinkled with delightful song parodies.

~Dr. Sam Bierstock, MD, BSEE, author Full Circle

Joan describes her depression very poignantly, and her personality shows through in every chapter. Her story is an important reminder not just of obtaining informed consent, but of the bias that mental health conditions and side effects are less important than physical conditions and physical side effects. When dealing with something acutely life-threatening like cancer, I understand the bias, but it is important to always take a good mental health history.

~Ariel Tabachnik, MD, Galynker Family Center for Bipolar Disorder

Joan and I met several years ago when she was tirelessly raising funds to bring her debut off-Broadway show, *Signs of Life*, to the stage. Her unwavering passion for getting this important production off the ground left a lasting impression on me. Imagine my delight when our paths converged again—a few years later—when Joan became a snowbird in Florida. I wasted no time inviting her to join the board of the Yiddishkayt Initiative. Joan infuses everything she does with boundless passion and energy. Her memoir is a powerful testament to the pursuit of one's dreams and the unwavering commitment to following one's passions.

~ Avi Hoffman, Founder/CEO of Yiddishkayt Initiative
and renowned Jewish cultural activist

All of the qualities I most admire in Joan—her sense of humor, her unstinting honesty, and her bone-deep love of musical theater—flourish in this memoir. We are treated to the fullness of her fantastic life, one that has paired uncommon inner resilience with a devoted communitarian spirit. Joan's journey will stay with and inspire you, as it has me.

--Susan Papp Lippman, co-adapter of Joe Papp
at the Ballroom (Gable Stage)

What a match! It was made by my daughter who said "Mom, I have someone you should meet…" and thus began a wonderful creative collaboration and friendship. As Joan recounts and examines the many obstacles life has thrown at her, you can't help but be inspired by the guts, resilience, and perseverance that accompany her immense talent. Her book is a terrific journey into the life of someone who, despite every difficult challenge, triumphs!

~ *Debbie Slevin, author, theatrical producer/director*

As I devoured this memoir, I found myself simultaneously nodding in agreement, gasping in anguish, laughing, and ultimately smiling. Bravo, Joan! This book invites the reader along for a deeply revealing story of those familiar moments of family, work, love, and loss, as well as those experiences that put our lives on pause such as bouts with depression and cancer. Joan's has been a life fully lived and through it all she has maintained a wonderfully contagious wit, humor, and perspective. This book is well-written, refreshingly honest, and both intimate and relatable. Readers will want to hug the author, sit down with her for a stimulating conversation over chocolate and wine, and… thank her.

~*Robert Watson Ph.D., Distinguished Professor of American History*

My LimanAde Life

A Story Of Relentless Resiliency

Joan Liman, MD

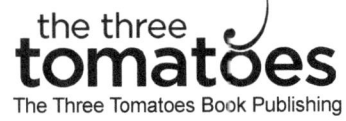

The Three Tomatoes Book Publishing

©2024 Joan Liman

All rights reserved. No part of this book may be reproduced in
any form or by any electronic or mechanical means, including
information storage and retrieval systems, without permission
in writing from the publisher. The only exception is by a reviewer,
who may quote short excerpts in a review.
For permission requests, please address
The Three Tomatoes Publishing.

Published January 2025

ISBN: 979-8-9903014-6-7
Library of Congress Control Number: 2024914043

For information address:
The Three Tomatoes Book Publishing
6 Soundview Road, Glen Cove, NY 11542

Photo: From the author's personal photos
Cover and interior design: Susan Herbst

All trademarks, service marks, and company names
are the property of their respective owners.

This work depicts actual events in the life of the author as
truthfully as recollection permits and/or can be verified by research.
Occasionally, dialogue consistent with the character
or nature of the person speaking has been supplemented.
All persons within are actual individuals; there are no composite
characters. The names of some individuals have been changed
to respect their privacy.

Dedication

My LimanAde Life is dedicated to my husband, Larry,
my daughter, Melanie, and my grandchildren,
Ryan and Marissa, as well as all those who inspired
and helped me to live it. As they say at the Tony Awards,
"You know who you are."

Table of Contents

Prologue

"Life can only be understood by looking backward; but it must be lived looking forward."

~Soren Kierkegaard (1813-1855)

The *Cambridge Dictionary* defines the noun *imponderable* as follows: Something that cannot be guessed or calculated because it is completely unknown. It gives the following example: There are too many imponderables to make an accurate forecast.

Personally, I think the sentiment written on my favorite refrigerator magnet is a better one: If we can send a man to the moon, why can't we send all of them?

Now and then I find myself contemplating real-life enigmas that range from the mundane to the metaphysical.

Why should I bother to wash bath towels? They're clean when I go into the shower and I'm clean when I come out.

Why does lipstick so easily wear off my lips when it seems to stick to my teeth forever?

How come my hearing-impaired husband can't seem to detect my voice when I am standing within close range but can hear my farts from clear across a room?

Its corollary, as inscribed on a cocktail napkin advertising Honey Nut Cheerios: *Nobody told me that when you get a husband the ears are sold separately.*

When I tell him the TV remote doesn't seem to be working, why does he pout and say, "What did you do to it?"

When I first moved to Florida from New Jersey, why was I so intimidated by self-service gas stations and why am I still flummoxed when I try to leave a NYC subway station whose only exit is a turnstile patterned after a Torquemada-style torture device dating back to the Inquisition?

Why do cell phones of people in theaters and at the movies go off so often despite the oft-repeated pre-curtain admonition to turn them off? (Probably because they belong to folks over the age of fifty-five who need a preschooler to help shut them down.)

You know you're getting old when you buy an eight-pack of condolence cards at Walgreens along with your recurring prescription for Lipitor and use both up within a month.

It sucks that cremation is the only surefire and pain-free way to achieve a smokin' hot body.

When I rinse soda cans out before recycling them, why do I feel compelled to crush them before tossing them into the bin? (Actually, this sounds more like a question for my therapist than an imponderable.)

Why is it called "common sense" when it is so rare?

If, as the Bible teaches, one of God's most miraculous acts was taking a rib from Adam to create Eve, why do his most devout adherents believe transsexualism is sinful?

How is it that the United States is the wealthiest country in the world, yet 37.9 million Americans are living in poverty?

How come doctors have twice the suicide rate as the general population?

Why do bad things happen to good people?

This last one is actually the title of a poignant book by Rabbi Harold Kushner, first published in 1981. (Not to be confused with 2009's *When Good Things Happen to Bad People* by Martin Levinson, an entirely different kettle of fish. Google it.) Coincidentally, 1981 was the same year a very bad thing happened to me.

However, I didn't become aware of Kushner's book until several years later when I was doing research for a presentation I had been asked to give at my synagogue. I learned Rabbi Kushner had started to question his faith in God when told his first child Aaron had been born with progeria, a disease of premature aging, which causes sufferers to die in their early teens. The diagnosis was made the very same day his second child—a healthy daughter—was born. Aaron died two days after his fourteenth birthday. Kushner writes about this paradox as follows:

> I don't know why one person gets sick and another does not, but I can only assume that some natural laws which we don't understand are at work. I don't believe in a God who has a weekly quota of malignant tumors to distribute and consults his computer to find out who deserves one most or who could handle it best. "What did I do to deserve this?" is an understandable outcry from a sick and suffering person but it is really the wrong question. The better question is "If this has happened to me, what do I do now and who is there to help me?"
>
> ~Harold S. Kushner, Why Bad Things Happen to Good People
> (published 2004 Anchor).

Reading these words resonated with me. Looking back at the many obstacles I had dealt with over the course of my life, I realized I had posed the same question to myself many times over and had, in fact, come up with an answer that enabled me to not only survive but thrive. I would like to share it with you by sharing the story of my "LimanAde life."

Introduction

Hello, my name is Joan, and I am a recovering academic. It's been more than twenty years since I chaired a faculty committee, conducted a literature search, or disciplined an unruly student. How did I go from "associate dean" to "being demeaned"? Let me set the stage.

A sunny spring morning in 2001 at New Jersey Medical School (NJMS) on the Newark campus of what was then named UMDNJ (University of Medicine and Dentistry of NJ)*. I had been employed as associate dean for Student Affairs since January 1993. I was in a great mood because a few days before, I'd been notified I had won a Golden Apple, a coveted award given by the student body. Winners are announced at the school's yearly spring formal, which was coming up in two weeks, so I'd been mentally running through my closet trying to decide what to wear. And I'd just returned from a wonderful weekend in Ontario at the annual meeting of student affairs officers from medical schools in the northeast US and Canada.

After seven years as a member, I had developed warm friendships with several of them, including my counterpart from University of Medicine and Dentistry of New Jersey's (UMDNJ) Robert

Wood Johnson Medical School, Susan Rosenthal, MD. As the organization's president that year, Susan was in charge of planning the agenda for the meeting. I had lobbied her to include some entertainment in the final session and offered to write and perform a song parody for it. Luckily, my performance was a hit.

I basked in my colleagues' rave reviews and requests for an encore at next year's meeting. So much so, I spent the return flight scribbling possibilities for future lyrics on the Air Canada cocktail napkins that accompanied each of my three celebratory glasses of wine—a personal best for me since chocolate is my go-to addiction. (Give me a box of Lindt truffles over a bottle of Chardonnay any day.)

But my good mood was brought to an abrupt halt as soon as I stepped into my office on Monday morning. "The dean called. Said he needs to see you as soon as you arrive," my secretary, Phyllis, informed me before I even put my pocketbook away. This was the first time I was ever summoned to his, or any other dean's, office in my entire academic career either as a student or employee. "OK, Phyllis, tell him I'm on my way." And so I walked down the hall, totally unaware that the incredible high generated by my Canadian performance was about to be shattered by a man recruited from Canada to succeed the recently retired NJMS dean.

I have decided not to refer to him by his real name here to avoid a defamation lawsuit should this memoir become available at fine bookstores everywhere. That is if you can find a fine bookstore anywhere these days—but that's a different story. For now, let's just stick with my story.

What you are about to read started off as a semi-autobiographical play incorporating parodies of my favorite pop and Broadway show tunes as well as some original songs. I successfully pitched it as "a little musical comedy about life's big tragedies" to various nonprofit organizations as well as theater festivals. That was no longer a viable strategy once the rapid outbreak of COVID-19 caused live theaters to shut down. To cope with the ensuing stress of the pandemic and stave off depression (a condition to which I am genetically predisposed), I decided to turn the play into a musical memoir. To reflect its theatrical genesis, I added well-known song titles from the musical theater canon as well as the American songbook at the start of every chapter to capture the gist of each one. Throughout the book, I incorporated excerpts from the score of the play, some of which were written to original music composed by me or a collaborator.

I hope my memoir will serve as an intangible legacy for my daughter and grandchildren and impart advice that will serve them well long after I'm gone: when tragedy strikes, don't be defined in it, find the divine in it. Which is just a more highfalutin way of saying, "When life gives you lemons, make lemonade." Or in my case, throw in a twist of lime and create "LimanAde."

In 2013, Rutgers University absorbed most of UMDNJ in what was then the largest academic merger in US history. The medical school in Newark is now known as Rutgers New Jersey Medical School.

Chapter 1

Broadway Lullaby

Song: "Lullaby of Broadway," sung by Jerry Orbach*

I didn't start out as a Liman. I made my debut on the world stage as Joan Pamela Rubenfeld. The setting: Maimonides Medical Center in Brooklyn, NY. The time: February 23, 1949, in the midst of a blizzard. This is most likely an omen that my life is destined to be filled with Sturm und Drang but until I reach adulthood, my life is remarkably unremarkable—except for one thing: my penchant for musical theater.

Ever since my mother took me to see my first Broadway show – *Fanny* – at age six – I was hooked. During play dates at the home of my friends from around the corner, the Werner sisters, I spent most of the time seated at their piano, using my index finger to plink out theme songs from our favorite TV shows.

When my mother, learned of this development from Mrs. Werner, she was delighted. She grew up listening to opera and desperately wanted to learn how to play the piano, but pianos and music lessons were not the norm for the children growing up in her impoverished neighborhood. So, it was only natural that my mother wanted her "Joanie" to have what she couldn't.

She convinced my father, Leon, to buy an upright piano that barely fit into the dining room of our row house on Homecrest Avenue, located on the border of Graves End and Sheepshead Bay. Then she set out to find a piano teacher.

Her search turned up Mr. Dupont, a slight, soft-spoken middle-aged gentleman whom, had I known the word at the time, I would have described as effete. He arrived impeccably dressed for my weekly lessons, sporting a stylish fedora and shirts with French cuffs to set off his bespoke suits. A gentle soul but a demanding instructor, he took out his metronome as soon as he sat down on one of our plastic-wrapped chairs and placed it on our mock-Italian provincial dining room table. The relentless ticking accompanied me as I "tickled" the ivories.

But mastering Bach fugues and Beethoven sonatas were not the accomplishments I was aiming for. I longed to learn theater tunes like "Oh, What a Beautiful Mornin'" and "I Could Have Danced All Night." Plus pop melodies such as the hit single "Diana," which topped the charts the year I become Mr. Dupont's pupil and turned me into a lifelong fan of Paul Anka.

So, Mr. Dupont and I struck a deal. If I demonstrated sufficient mastery of the classical canon, he would reward me each month with a piece of contemporary sheet music. Ever the overachiever, I diligently practiced my scales and arpeggios and studied music theory. Eventually, complete scores from Tony Award-winning shows coupled with a compendium of theme songs from Elvis Presley movies began to compete with Mozart concertos for storage space inside the maroon-brocaded piano bench.

On the rare occasions when I had the house all to myself (which wasn't very often since my mother rarely went anywhere except for grocery shopping and my father was away on business for weeks at a time), I belted out lyrics like an a pint-sized Ethel Merman to my self-accompaniment. At first, I would stick to the easy-to-play standards such as "Let Me Entertain You" from Gypsy, considered to be the best Broadway musical ever written. Music by Jule Styne, lyrics by Stephen Sondheim and book by Arthur Laurents. Need I say more?

Mind you, it was not until I saw the big screen movie version with Rosalind Russell that I realized it was actually the theme song for the title character, the famous stripper Gypsy Rose Lee. Then my signature song switched to *Flower Drum Song's* breakout hit, "I Enjoy Being a Girl." And by the time I entered JHS 234 (aka Cunningham Junior High School, I really did.

Fun Fact: Jerry Orbach was a musical comedy star long before Law and Order!

Chapter 2

The Pastina Legacy

Song: "Memory" sung by Betty Buckley

"I think it's time to introduce some solid food into Melanie's diet," announced Dr. Wolmer at my daughter's three-month checkup in the winter of 1972. "Try some pastina."

Pastina—those tiny, star-shaped pieces of pasta that spill out all over the kitchen counter if you don't pry open the cardboard package just so. I hadn't heard that product mentioned in at least fifteen years when our pediatrician prescribed it for my newborn baby. The mention of it brought back a flood of memories involving my mother, many of which were painful because they tended to revolve around her lifelong struggle with depression.

Up until I heard the term "nature vs. nurture" in my first college psychology course, I just assumed the foundation for my mother's condition was laid down early in her life based on what I had gleaned about her from family lore.

Her parents—Sophie and Gershon—were born in Eastern Europe where they met, married, and had several children. At least one of the children passed away before the family emigrated to the United States around the turn of the century. (Supposedly he was mischievously rocking back and forth on a chair, fell off, hit his head, and died—a fate that seems to have morphed into a cautionary urban legend still prevalent today in parenting circles.)

Their youngest child, Ruth Lillian Goodman, was my mother. She had three brothers—Morris, Louis, and Jack—and two sisters—Dorothy and Sylvia. Ruth was a change of life baby. Seven years separated her from Sylvia, and her oldest brother Morris was already a father when Ruth was born in Brooklyn in 1914.

The Goodmans grew up in poverty as did many of the families in their Williamsburg neighborhood. But my grandfather's "nervous" condition hampered his ability to earn money, though what he actually did for a living was never made clear. "Selling antiques" was the term I heard bandied about but, in reality, he was probably a junk dealer. Had the internet and antidepressants existed back then, he might have made a killing on eBay or Craigslist while popping Paxil or Wellbutrin without ever having to leave home.

Sadly, he died when Ruth was six years old. So essentially, she became an only child being raised by an elderly mother whose three sons and eldest daughter helped Sophie and the two youngest children to stay afloat. And even though she was a first generation American, Ruth spoke only Yiddish until she started school. The isolation and loneliness growing up in a poor, fatherless household had an indelible effect on my mother, and no doubt resulted in her seeking a father figure to be her mate. Enter Leon Rubenfeld, whose backstory was almost a mirror image of hers.

Leon was the eldest of five children born in 1911 to Austrian-born Abraham Rubenfeld and Sarah Rubin, American-born and bred. After him came Eleanor, Paul, Florence, and Murray in quick succession. My paternal grandfather was a glazier, installing and repairing windows and mirrors in the same neighborhood where the Goodman family resided.

The Rubins were better off financially and more acculturated than the Rubenfelds so Sarah's station in life was lowered when she married Abraham. She was not used to having to worry about money and this may have contributed to a nervous breakdown for which she was briefly hospitalized.

She died when my father was seventeen, leaving him to "mother" his four siblings. He went to work immediately after graduating high school and took college classes at night but dropped out after six months because of the burden of being both a student and caretaker for his family.

My parents met when they were teenagers and married in 1935. My mother had a hard time conceiving so my sister, Susan, didn't come along until six years later; another eight years passed until I entered the world on a snowy February 23, 1949.

Grandma Sophie lived with us at 2213 Homecrest Avenue, our one-family home in Sheepshead Bay. She prepared most of the meals, so my mother never really learned how to cook. We "kept kosher" at home in deference to my grandmother but most Sunday nights found us happily dining on barbecued spareribs and chow mein at the local Chinese restaurant on Avenue U. On special occasions, we splurged for lobster at Lundy's Seafood, a Brooklyn institution for generations of secular Jews.

Sadly, Sophie passed away when I was still a toddler, and I don't really have any memories of her. What I do recall is that after her death, a package of bacon made its first appearance in our refrigerator and to this day, it is one of my favorites (but calorically verboten) foods.

Which brings me back to pastina, the comfort food of my childhood. During my elementary school years, on days when I felt too sick to go to class but not sick enough to be confined to my bed, my mother would prepare a steaming hot bowl of pastina for me as soon as I woke up. To enhance its bland taste, she liberally laced it with butter and salt, cholesterol and hypertension not yet having been demonized as medical taboos back in the mid-1950s.

As a special treat to compensate for having to miss a day or two of school (yes, I confess I was one of those handkerchief-bearing, saddle shoe-wearing teacher's pets who actually loved being in the classroom and hated to fall behind in my work by staying home), my mother would allow me to take the bowl into our living room and slurp down my breakfast pasta while cozily ensconced in the plastic-covered turquoise armchair that occupied the place of honor in front of the black-and-white RCA television set. There I'd sit from 9:00 a.m. to noon, watching all my favorite morning TV shows. *My Little Margie* with Gale Storm, *December Bride* with Spring Byington, and of course, *I Love Lucy* starring America's favorite real-life Hollywood couple, Lucille Ball and Desi Arnaz.

Lulled into somnolence by my carbohydrate-laden repast, I didn't have the attention span or focus for game shows that made up the afternoon programming of the major network channels of which there were three—CBS on Channel 2, NBC on Channel 4, and ABC on Channel 7. So, I would turn off the TV around noon and retreat to the spartan surroundings of my five-foot-by-eight-foot bedroom where I curled up and cocooned under the covers until my mother trudged up the stairs carrying a bowl of Campbell's chicken noodle soup accompanied by cellophane packages of saltine crackers and a glass of Dr. Brown's Cel-Ray soda on a worn, wooden tray. A one-inch stack of paper napkins was tucked under the bowl to wipe up the inevitable spills of soup and soda. After lunch, I would spend the rest of the day listening to audio soap operas on our Philco radio until I drifted off to sleep.

The warm memories of the days spent in Ruth's sick bay have remained firmly lodged in my mind. So, when Dr. Wolmer proposed that I introduce pastina as my daughter's first solid food, I was more than happy to comply. And Melanie was more than eager to eat it. To this day, pastina remains a favorite comfort food for her as well as her two children. And I still keep a package tucked in the far reaches of my cupboard to remind me that despite recollections of my mother's chronic bouts of mental illness, I also have memories tinged with a pleasant aura to remind me of the warmth and love she had for me throughout her life.

Chapter 3

The Saltwater Cure

Song: "By the Beautiful Sea," sung by Julie London

The birth of my only sibling, Susan, triggered my mother's first episode of depression. When I came along eight years later, Susan got to witness the second one firsthand. As it turned out, Ruth's mood disorder was more than just a postpartum thing. I was reluctant to bring friends to play at our house after school for fear she would still be in her nightgown, wringing her hands and pacing the floor. And though my father taught her how to drive, she was too frightened to get behind the wheel without him beside her. We lived in Brooklyn, so this didn't pose too much of a problem since everything she needed to run a home was within short walking distance.

Still, I envied my friends whose mothers took them ice skating in Prospect Park, swimming at Brighton Beach, and ferried them to after school clubs and activities. And I still remember how crestfallen I was at the beginning of third grade in PS 153 when she wouldn't let me join the Brownies. Oh, how I yearned to wear the coffee-colored uniform, with its shiny sash slung across my chest and a brown felt beanie perched atop my head. But being a Brownie meant your mother had to get involved in the troop's activities as well. And that was simply out of the question for Ruth. "Joanie, you know that would be too stressful for my nerves."

Third grade also remains memorable in my mind because that was the one and only time my father, Leon, ever set foot inside PS 153. His name at birth was Leo but my mother thought it wasn't refined enough and insisted he go by Leon.

Leon was a "garmento" employed as a traveling salesman by Columbia Dance Frocks, a modest-size company in the middle of Manhattan's Garment District. Our Chrysler sedan was fitted with an iron bar over the back seat; from it hung the satiny, lace-bedecked samples of wedding gowns and bridesmaid dresses he peddled to large department stores as well as mom-and-pop specialty shops from Baltimore to Buffalo and throughout New England. His work required him to be on the road for two to three weeks at a time.

When he was home, his time was taken up paying the bills that had accumulated in his absence. Back then, such activities were pretty much considered a de facto responsibility of the male of the house and my mother was more than happy to keep it that way *chez* Rubenfeld.

So, when my father showed up in Mrs. Siegel's third-grade classroom on a Thursday afternoon in early April, when he was supposed to be in Boston, I was shocked. We'd just finished our weekly music instruction on the tonette, a sort of mini recorder designed to prepare us for more formal music training in fourth grade. As I looked up from my desk, I saw my father standing in front of Mrs. Siegel, his back toward me. I squirmed around in my seat to try to see what was going on between them.

Suddenly, Mrs. Siegel clapped her hands to silence the whispered buzzing of my classmates and announced, "Joan, please gather your belongings and go with your father. We'll see you back here on Monday."

I felt my face redden as I did what I was told. I made my way from the last seat in the fifth row (compliments of my last name falling at the end of the alphabet) to the front of the classroom. He took my hand, and we proceeded down the hallway and outside to the school yard—the same yard that had been teeming with the noisy sounds of children at recess only one hour earlier but was now eerily silent as we walked through to get to the trusty Chrysler.

Once inside, he put his arm around me and with what I now realize was forced cheerfulness, announced he had a surprise. "I'm taking you, Mommy, and Susan to Atlantic City for a special weekend vacation."

"But Daddy, Easter isn't 'til the end of April. Why are we going away now? Won't the ocean be too cold for us to go swimming?"

"Well, you know Mommy isn't a very strong lady and sometimes it's hard for her to take care of you and Susan all by herself, especially when I am away at work. It makes her nervous and when she feels like that, she gets agitated and upset."

"Is that why she sometimes screams at us?"

"Uh-huh. And even hits you."

"Mostly Susan." Like when Susan hangs out with boys my mother calls "hoodlum goys"—aka non-Jewish kids from the neighborhood with last names like Abruzzi or O'Reilly. Almost all of them attend Grady Vocational, the high school across the street from hers—Abraham Lincoln—alma mater of Arthur Miller, Neil Sedaka, and other accomplished alumni.

"Susan called me yesterday and said Mommy has been especially upset while I've been away these past three weeks. She's been very tired and doesn't seem to have energy to do the things she needs to do for you and your sister while I'm on the road."

"Is that why she's been staying in bed so much each day? And why she gets angry when I try to pull off the covers and ask her to play with me?"

He pulled me closer to him and kissed the top of my head.

"Yes, Joanie. It's not that she doesn't love you. She's just sick right now; her doctor says it would be good for her to spend some time away from the house. Somewhere near the ocean. He says the sea air cures everything."

Excitedly I asked, "You mean like Coney Island?"

To me, Coney Island was nirvana. The fun house with its body-morphing mirrors, the whiplash-inducing bumper cars, the coveted, always slightly out-of-reach brass ring and the ginormous Ferris wheel whose cars whisk you up, down, and around while simultaneously sliding back and forth on a sort of high wire. This attraction is certainly worthy of its name—the Wonder Wheel. And of course, there's the dizzying array of eponymous carny food: Nathan's sizzling hot dogs and crinkly French fries, Mrs. Stahl's delicious knishes with a variety of fillings (potato, spinach, even chopped liver) and an Orange Julius to wash everything down.

But the primary reason I was so enthralled with Brooklyn's most famous beach attraction is that I had my father all to myself on the rare Sundays he was able to indulge in a carefree excursion there because he was not traveling. My sister had long since outgrown the honky-tonk seediness of the place, preferring to spend weekends at the movies with her teenaged friends. As for my mother, well she never once accompanied my father and me on these or any other outings, claiming she'd had a very stressful week and needed some time alone to calm her nerves. Interestingly enough though, on those occasions when she'd reached what seemed to be her breaking point, she threatened to drown herself at Coney Island.

So, it was quite ironic her doctor had prescribed a long weekend at the seashore to lift her spirits. But my eight-year-old brain had not yet learned to process irony. It was too busy free-associating images of being at the beach and the happy times I spent there with my father. My reverie was interrupted by the sound of my father's voice.

"Even better, Joanie. Atlantic City."

"Where's that?"

"New Jersey. You know that beauty contest you and Susan like to watch every September? What's it called?"

"The Miss America Pageant."

"That's the one. It's held in a big auditorium called Convention Hall. We can go visit it. I bet there's probably a room where you can see pictures and costumes from each year's pageant. That would be fun, right?"

"Is there a boardwalk?"

"Uh-huh. With rolling cars that a whole family can ride in from one end of it to the other. And there are twice as many food stands along it as there are in Coney Island. Plus, a very famous candy that's made in Atlantic City. It's called Fralinger's Salt Water Taffy, and it comes in all sorts of flavors."

"Chocolate?"

"Of course. Well, it's settled there," my dad reassured me. "As soon as we get to Atlantic City, I will buy you the biggest box of salt water taffy we can find." He put the key in the ignition, started the car and drove the two blocks that separated our two-story attached house from the school.

My mother and Susan were already waiting on our front porch, suitcases at their feet. My father and Susan put the suitcases in the trunk, but my mother remained rooted where she was. Finally, at my dad's urging, she started to walk down the front steps at a snail's pace, making it look like she was in slow motion.

Later on, I came to discover that the apple didn't fall far from the maternal tree when I experienced my first episode of depression and exhibited the same psychomotor retardation—the clinical term for my mother's behavior on the steps that blustery April afternoon. I learned that it is a common sign of clinical depression. The opposite kind of behavior can also occur. A depressed person may be unable to sit still and wring his or her hands while pacing back and forth, almost like an automaton. I have seen my mother in both of these states and experienced them myself and still can't decide which one is preferable.

But at the moment, a little urgency in her stride would have been nice because my father was impatiently honking the horn. Like the lyrics of that Willie Nelson standard, he longs "to be back on the road again."

Chapter 4

You Can Go Home Again…
But It Probably Won't Look the Same

Song: "Summer in the City" sung by the Lovin' Spoonful

Sunday, August 8, 2021, 5:30 a.m.

It **was pitch-black as I** pulled out of my garage and turned left to begin the ninety-mile drive to Monticello, a town located in New York's Sullivan County, aka the Catskills. I was headed to the town's annual Bagelfest, a street fair with vendors and organizations ranging from the local head shop to national health insurance companies.

I had to be at 275 Main Street by 7:30 a.m. to set up an exhibit for Yiddishkayt Initiative (YI), a not-for-profit organization based in Coral Springs, Florida. My husband and I had purchased a condo in nearby Boca Raton some twenty years before while both of us were still working full-time. Initially, we were "snowflakes" escaping the cold winters of New Jersey from time to time as our schedules would allow. Gradually we transitioned to "snowbirds," spending summers up north and wintering in Palm Beach County.

Since I've never been a golfer and spinal surgery at the age of sixty-eight put an end to playing tennis, I sought out a sedentary pastime to keep me busy during retirement. Given my interests in the arts and my Jewish heritage, YI seemed a perfect fit since its mission is to battle anti-Semitism through the arts by celebrating and promoting Jewish history, life, and culture and their positive, far-reaching impact on the world. I started volunteering in April 2019 and joined the board of directors soon thereafter.

After about a year I was asked to take on the role of acting Chief Operating Officer, albeit unpaid. As one of the goals is to increase the awareness of the organization and build brand recognition, we strive to maintain a healthy presence on social media. But since I'm an "analog person in a digital world," I still think on-the-ground, in-your-face grassroots marketing is the best way to recruit potential customers and sponsors to a cause.

This is why I'd signed up to staff a booth at Bagelfest 2021. Waze had my ETA at 7:05 a.m.; my internal GPS said the trip would take me backward to the summer of 1959, the last time I was there. I was curious to see the changes that had taken place in the interim.

Back then, many Jewish families from the five boroughs of New York and the outlying suburbs sought the lush greenery of the Catskill Mountains to escape the "hot town, summer in the city" days of July and August. They flocked to towns like Monticello, Loch Sheldrake, and Kiamesha Lake where lodgings ran the gamut from high-rise hotels with luxury suites and fancy gift shops to *kuchelains*—modest bungalow colonies where families shared a common kitchen and peddlers traveled from one to the other hawking a variety of wares. (Think *A Walk on the Moon*, that wonderful movie starring Diane Lane and Viggo Mortenson). My family wasn't sufficiently well-heeled to afford a stay at The Concord or Grossinger's, but we were flush enough to check into a more upscale locale than a bungalow colony, only because we took one room for the four of us and our length of stay was never more than four weeks. Our summer home away from home was a medium-sized hotel called the Greenwood Inn, located in Ellenville, NY.

Preparations for our departure began around the second week of June. My father would lug the two-foot-by-five-foot-by-two-and-a-half-foot black steamer trunk up from the basement and deposit it in our living room. Believe it or not, almost the entire vacation wardrobe for the family had to fit in that one piece of luggage because my mother thought it was tacky to strap suitcases on the roof of our car. She didn't want fellow travelers to think my father was driving a "hack"—the name given to taxis shared by strangers who didn't own their own cars. (No surprise as this is the same woman who made my father change his name from Leo to Leon because it sounded classier. While he never made it legal, I didn't learn his given name until I brought home some paperwork from junior high school that required both parents' signatures.)

Leon would position the well-worn trunk between the marble-topped coffee table and the plastic-covered brocade couch, rendering the only room in the house with a TV practically inaccessible until it was time to take off. The lid would stay open and every day, my mother would add more articles of clothing, the fabric and style of which were designed to accommodate scorching heat waves as well as Arctic temperatures. ("It gets cold in the mountains at night. You never know when you might need a parka and earmuffs. Or mink stole.")

A hat-boxed piece of luggage containing toiletries, makeup, and medicines was the third back seat passenger between my sister and me. A few of our favorite evening dresses plus my father's best suit were sheathed in plastic garment bags, courtesy of my father's occupation. They hung from the same hooks on either side of the rear windows that held the sample bridal wear he took on his out-of-town trips to department stores and retail shops.

Eventually, Kodachrome slides of the inventory replaced the actual garments but by then the strain from years of schlepping billowing wedding gowns with four-foot trains and bead-encrusted cocktail dresses had taken its toll on my dad's back. He developed severe sciatica in his late fifties, causing him to take early retirement from a job he loved and had earned him the respect and admiration of his colleagues.

When I was still in elementary school, he would sometimes take me with him to the company's Seventh Avenue showroom and treat me to lunch at nearby Dubrow's Cafeteria, a longtime fixture in the neighborhood. As we walked the three short blocks, I was awestruck by all the people who greeted him by name, slapped him on the back, and exchanged pleasantries. No wonder I idolized my dad and made him my role model rather than my same-sex parent, whose world had become narrowly circumscribed once she became a bride.

She didn't go to college and only spent a brief period of time working in an office as a bookkeeper before she had my sister. She didn't do volunteer work, belong to Hadassah, or join the PTA—all outlets that would have afforded her the opportunity to socialize with other women. And then there was the whole question of transporting me to after-school activities. Though my father taught her to drive, she was too nervous to get on the road, so she depended on him to take her to any places that weren't within walking distance of our house. That's why she wasn't able to share the driving during our seasonal journey.

But my father didn't seem to mind. After all, he was used to being alone in the car for hours at a time when he was working; now he had a captive audience and he took advantage of the opportunity, transforming into a sort of tour guide pointing out various milestones along the way. When the car emerged out of the blackness of the Brooklyn-Battery Tunnel into the sunlit canyons of lower Manhattan, he'd let out a whoop of accomplishment. "Hip, hip, hooray," he'd bellow to signify that we'd left our everyday life in Brooklyn behind and were well on our way to the fun and excitement that now lay a mere three hours away.

The next marker was our lunch stop at the Red Apple Rest. As he pulled off Route 17 into the parking lot, he sternly reminded us it would be the last pit stop before we reached our final destination. The restaurant had a rustic ambience with a menu that appealed to the taste buds of its many city-bred patrons – sort of Cracker Barrel crossed with the Carnegie Deli. The place is still in existence but now the New York State Thruway parallels Route 17, offering a much quicker route to upstate NY. Those in search of a bit of nostalgia to break up the monotony of high-speed highways and cookie-cutter rest stops would do well to take a side trip to this iconic landmark.

Our bladders emptied and our bellies full, my father would herd us back in the car for the final leg of our journey. Soon, huge billboards emblazoned with the names of all sorts of lodgings began to dot the landscape, each one trying to outdo the other in their claims of excellence: Homowack Lodge—Indoor Ice Skating Rink and so forth.

Greenwood Inn, "owned and operated by the Buchholz Family," boasted no special amenities to speak of but did have everything my family required for a luxury stay in the mountains—comfortable lodgings, all-you-can eat meals, outdoor pool, and nightly entertainment in the "casino" with special shows on the weekends featuring comics, singers, ballroom dancers, and other performers making the rounds of the Borscht Belt's night clubs.

For me, the best feature was the hotel's day camp that sat nestled in a hollow facing the pool, surrounded by towering trees. It was just a short stroll down a gently sloping hill from the children's dining room, a nondescript building that nevertheless evoked powerful memories. It wasn't because of the decor or the food, neither of which was anything to write home about. No, it was the unique smells that emanated from it.

This isn't surprising considering that smell is the sense most tied to memory. Our olfactory receptor neurons, which are located behind our sinuses and are the only neurons in the body exposed to air, make physical contact with whatever molecules compose an odor. Then they instantly send that info straight to the brain. Our sense of smell is so strong that it aids dramatically in how we perceive taste, even going as far as affecting our behavior, emotions, perceptions, and memories, more so than any of our other senses.

Researchers hypothesize that the exceptional ability that smells have to trigger memories—known as the Proust effect—is due to how close the olfactory processing system is to the memory hub in the brain. To put it another way: "Seeing vomit might make you want to throw up but smelling vomit is what ultimately triggers your gag reflex."

My equivalent of Proust's madeleine is the seductive sweetness of U-Bet chocolate syrup used to create the calorie-laden chocolate milk available at breakfast wafting alongside the aromatic pungency of onions being sautéed to mix into the kosher chopped meat that will be transformed into well-done hamburgers for lunch. Forget about ordering your burger rare or even medium; or downing it with a big cold glass of the aforementioned chocolate milk.

Thanks to the dictates of kashruth, such culinary choices are not an option in the Catskills hotels catering to Jews. For example: milk can't be mixed with meat and meat must be cooked to the consistency of shoe leather. It wasn't until I was well into my twenties after seeing *American Graffiti* that I defied either of these commandments and discovered the culinary thrill of a rare cheeseburger paired with a black-and-white ice cream soda chaser. (Thank you, Ron Howard).

Day camp left a lasting impression on my other senses. I can still visualize the rustic bunkhouse that served as the sleeping quarters for the counselors and the unisex washroom, which was more like an indoor outhouse, with a variety of insects—dead and alive—festooning the walls. There was also a large all-purpose room used during inclement weather where we would spend the time playing team games like dodgeball and steal the bacon. The latter was one of the most popular pastimes despite its nonkosher title.

My favorite activity was the Saturday camp show held in the poolside clubhouse. I was always relegated to the chorus but managed to snag some lines when I was cast as one of the ladies-in-waiting in *The King and I*. My costume was a white terry cloth hotel towel wrapped around me like a sarong, decorated with strips of brightly colored crepe paper and a "pearl" necklace made of white plastic pop-it beads, a fashion accessory that was all the rage that summer of 1961, the last one I would spend at Greenwood Inn.

In the late spring of that year my mother was told she needed a hysterectomy. This was back when such operative procedures involved a weeklong hospitalization followed by a prescribed period of post-op bed rest. My parents decided it would be best to schedule it for the beginning of the summer so that my father could take me on the road with him while my sister, who was in high school by then, stayed home to look after my mother.

So, off we went that July, an odd traveling couple to say the least. I was a head taller than most of my classmates and had started to develop breasts long before most of them, a turn of events that mortified me. Since I was slated to start junior high school that fall, my mother told my father it was his job to ensure that by the time we returned from our travels, I had traded in all the white cotton undershirts I had packed in my suitcase for the nylon training bras she had hidden away in his. And though most of the time he was able to secure a motel room with one bed for each of us, there were a few occasions when we pulled into a sleepy little town late at night after a long day's drive and the only available accommodation was a room with a double bed.

While I might have appeared mature for my age, no doubt some of the desk clerks must have looked at us askance as they handed over the room keys. I, of course, was oblivious to all this. I was so thrilled to have my father all to myself it never dawned on me that sleeping next to him might be construed as "inappropriate." And indeed, it wasn't. Within minutes after tucking me in and turning off the lights, he was snoring soundly, exhausted after a long day of hustling his wares.

That summer marked the first one we didn't vacation as a family in the Catskills. And we never did vacation there together ever again. My sister went off to college soon after and I preferred to hang out with my friends at Brighton Beach Baths, a city version of a suburban swim club bordering the Atlantic Ocean, easily reached by the BMT subway and within walking distance of Coney Island. Come to think of it, I haven't been back to that part of Brooklyn in a long while either, though I have equally fond memories of the summer months I spent there—riding the Cyclone, playing paddleball at Manhattan Beach, dining alfresco (i.e. on the sidewalk) at Mrs. Stahl's Knishes and viewing Tuesday night fireworks over the Atlantic.

Now the area is referred to as Little Odessa because of the influx of Russian immigrants that started arriving back in the 1970s. I hardly recognized the place when I went back to Brooklyn with my grandchildren to show them where Nonny had grown up. I took them to the aquarium and pointed out what passed for amusement parks before Walt Disney ever broke ground for his eponymous empire. Pierogies had replaced knishes and vodka flowed as freely as lemonade did when my father and I walked the boardwalk lined with carnival barkers hawking attractions like Whack a Mole. Little did I know then that I would co-opt that beverage and that game to describe the way my adult years would eventually unfold.

Chapter 5

Confessions of a
Seventh-Grade Stalker

Song: "I Will Follow Him" sung by Peggy March

Thank God my father heeded my mother's admonition to
bring me back from our summer sojourn wearing a bra. In our
absence, she'd received a letter from Cunningham JHS containing
important information for incoming seventh graders; one item described the required uniform for girls' gym class that turned out
to be a fitted, short-sleeved, bile-colored romper that resembled
an abbreviated version of a prison jumpsuit. It had to be stored in
similarly colored lockers lining the female changing room that did
not provide for any privacy while taking off our school clothes and
donning said uniform.

Since several elementary schools fed into Cunningham, I
would inevitably be in gym class with many girls I had never laid
eyes on before. The thought of them laying eyes on me wearing a
size extra-large Carter's white undershirt instead of a stretchy nylon training bra unnerved me because I knew I would be the subject
of their scorn and taunts. I allowed my mother to take me shopping
at the neighborhood undergarment store staffed by portly women

with blue-tinted hair, all of whom appeared to be not a day younger than dead. One of them shuffled over to me brandishing a tape measure as if it were a lasso, and roped me in "so we can find out our bust size."

"Our" size? What are we? Siamese twins joined at the rib cage? And why does she use the word *bust*? Does she think I am a teen-aged Jewish Jayne Mansfield? Apparently, she did because she announced I was too full-figured for a training bra and would be best served by getting one of those Playtex Cross Your Heart brassieres. Naturally, this freaked me out, but I softened my stance somewhat at the sight of the cute options she laid out before me and settled on a pretty lace-edged number. It came in a variety of colors, but my mother insisted on white—"it's the most practical"—and I didn't put up a fight. I even agreed to wear one out of the store, arms tightly crossed over my heart to hide my cleavage (pun intended).

In retrospect, I probably shouldn't have had such a negative reaction to the thought of being compared to Jayne Mansfield; after all, she was the mother of *Law and Order*'s Mariska Hargitay and was reported to speak five languages and have an IQ of 149. Though mine is not nearly as impressive, it was sufficient to gain entrance into the "SP"—NYC's special program for intellectually gifted adolescents, the baby-boomer-generation equivalent of a gifted and talented curriculum. As initially designed, it allowed qualified sixth graders to enroll in an accelerated junior high school track where three years were condensed into two by skipping eighth grade.

Around the time I became eligible for it, an alternative pathway sprung up as an option. Dubbed "the three-year SP," it did not shorten the junior high school length of stay; instead, it offered enrichment classes that were more rigorous than those of the traditional seventh, eighth, and ninth grade curricula. SP-eligible candidates who skipped a grade earlier in their elementary school careers often took this route as they were already among the youngest (and often smallest) kids in their grade. Leapfrogging yet another year ahead might put them at further social disadvantage. I was one of the oldest students in my grade, having missed the December 31 kindergarten entry cutoff date by a few weeks. So, I was chomping at the bit to truncate my formal education except for one drawback: Billy Wechsler, my very first boyfriend, skipped first grade and we would have to part ways since he would be taking the three-year SP.

I had no idea Billy even existed until he showed up in Mrs. Garbow's second-grade classroom. He attracted everyone's attention, but what really made him stand out were his bright red hair and matching freckles marching across his nose and cheeks. He was the first "ginger" I'd ever encountered, and I was fascinated. It was as if Ron Howard as Opie in *The Andy Griffith Show* had left Mayberry and taken up residence in Brooklyn. To add to his charm, Billy's quick wit and cunning intelligence made him seem like a cross between Dennis the Menace and Huckleberry Finn. Unfortunately, Mrs. Garbow wasn't as enamored with Billy as I was. A tiny, birdlike woman, she was not up to verbally sparring with him and wound up being a straight man to his routine. Since a sense of humor is a quality I'd come to appreciate despite my young age, this endeared him to me all the more.

Billy's January birthday made him eleven months my junior, but the age difference didn't dissuade me from considering him as a potential suitor. He didn't pick up on my vibes, but I was not that concerned. Thanks to the elementary school tracking placement system in use back in the "pre-woke" era of the fifties and sixties, Billy and I were destined to travel in tandem throughout our remaining years in PS 153. Grade size stayed pretty much constant so at any given time there were approximately 170 students distributed over five classes and the title of each class was a numerical designation based on academic standing, e.g., 2-1, 2-2, 2-3, etc.

Fast forward to fourth grade, where class 4-1 was presided over by Mrs. Devlin who was a lot more intimidating than any of her predecessors. A spunky redhead whose name reflected her demeanor, she was more than a match for Billy's antics. Maybe it was because they were both gingers that there were sparks between them. Her teaching style was in keeping with her personality. Mrs. D. was not content to let us learn things by rote; she challenged us to be critical thinkers.

Take her lesson plan on measurement. "What weighs more, a pound of feathers or a pound of bricks?" This seemed like a no-brainer, but only Billy failed to succumb to the pedagogical trap she had laid. "They both weigh the same." My classmates and I sat with mouths agape at his answer that seemed to fly in the face of our collective logic. "Their volume is different," he continued. "It takes a larger number of lightweight feathers to add up to a pound than it does dense, heavy bricks." His reply heightened my attraction to him. Even at the tender age of ten, I valued brains over brawn.

On the annual class trip aboard the Circle Line for a sightseeing tour around Manhattan, I made it my business to spend most of the three-hour cruise in his proximity. In fifth grade he invited me to do homework together at his house. In sixth grade, I spent more time with him after school during our weekly Hebrew school classes at Temple Beth El located on Avenue T between Homecrest Avenue and East Thirteenth Street, right around the corner from his house. With the passage of more time, it was apparent we'd become boyfriend and girlfriend.

Alas, the relationship began to unravel when we started seventh grade because of our respective SP tracks. They never coincided and since I had dropped out of Hebrew school because it conflicted with piano lessons, I'd lost the opportunity to see him outside of Temple Beth El. Here is where my tale of romance took a dark turn—I started to stalk him.

I went out of my way to walk or bike ride past his house hoping to bump into him. I could always use my friend Evelyn Mittleman as a cover because her house was down the block from Billy's, right off Avenue U. Evelyn and I had been best friends ever since the fall of fourth grade when she moved to Brooklyn from Yonkers. I still remember the outfit she was wearing when Mrs. Devlin introduced her to the class: navy blue skirt, white blouse, and red vest. When Mrs. Devlin asked for someone to help orient the newcomer to her new school and neighborhood, my hand quickly shot up before Barbara Ann Spector could volunteer. Barbara Ann lived one block closer to Evelyn, so I feared Mrs. Devlin would choose her. Luckily, I prevailed.

Evelyn and her older sister, Gwen, had moved to Brooklyn after their divorced mother married the neighborhood doctor whose office was on the bottom floor of his two-story house. Dr. Rossman had treated me years earlier after a bad fall from my bicycle required stitches. It was a very unpleasant medical encounter. He had a gruff demeanor and the bedside manner of a hit man. My impression was confirmed when Evelyn confided how badly her stepfather treated her. His son, Henry, was even worse. Periodically Evelyn sported a black eye because he had punched her or thrown her down the stairs.

I spent a lot of time at her house trying to soften the sadness of her home life (and to avoid spending time in the presence of my depressed mother, who rarely left the house). I was unlikely to arouse Billy's suspicion if I casually ran into him because I could always explain that I was either on my way to or just leaving Evelyn's.

Sadly, despite all my furtive skulking to reinsert myself into Billy's life, never once did it pay off. I came to feel like Charlie Brown in Charles Schultz's *Peanuts* comic strip, pining away for the little red-haired girl—only in my situation, the unrequited love was for a not-so-little red-haired boy. It was not until several months later that I discovered my sinister efforts had been for naught. Unbeknownst to me, shortly after starting seventh grade Billy took up with a blue-eyed, blond-haired vixen from one of the feeder schools. Even if my short career as a stalker had proved successful, it would not have made one bit of difference. Nevertheless, old habits die hard, and it wouldn't be the last time I would stoop so low to land a man.

Chapter 6

Mellow Yellow

Song: "Mellow Yellow" sung by Donovan

Pop Quiz*
Which of the following pathological conditions is most closely associated with the color yellow?

a. Oxygen deprivation

b. Purpura

c. Carbon monoxide poisoning

d. Hepatitis

Answer:

d. Hepatitis

I learned this years before I got to medical school.

The dog days of August 1963 were winding down; the start of tenth grade was less than a month away. Evelyn and I were shopping for school clothes at Charley Horse, the go-to store for teenage girls seeking the latest fashion trends by manufacturers such as John Meyer, The Villager, and Pappagallo. We spent an entire afternoon trying on button-down shirts, plaid skirts, and shoes to match. After a stop at the nearby pizza parlor for a slice and a vanilla Coke (total cost twenty-five cents), we headed to the Kings Highway subway station.

We took the BMT one stop to Avenue U. I bid her goodbye at East Thirteenth Street and continued the short walk to my house. Along the way I began to feel stomach cramps, so I quickened my pace, which wasn't easy since I was loaded down with shopping bags. Fortunately, I made it home just in time to make it to the bathroom. I emerged pale and sweaty to find my mother standing outside the door.

"I heard you come in at least ten minutes ago, Joanie. What's going on? You look awful. Your eyes are yellow and so is your skin." She placed her hand on my forehead then jerked it away as if she'd just touched a hot stove. "You're burning up. Go and lie down. I'll get the thermometer and meet you in your room."

I trudged upstairs, dragging my sore behind behind me. My mother soon appeared, thermometer in one hand, bottle of Bayer aspirin in the other. I glumly inserted the thermometer in my mouth while she went to get a glass of water from the bathroom. She set it down on my dresser and bustled about straightening up my room. After what seemed like an eternity, she removed it and announced, "I better go call Dr. Beecher. You have a fever of 102.8. Here, take two aspirin. Stay in bed and read." Before she exited she smiled good-naturedly. "You certainly have enough material to choose from."

I think I was genetically destined to become a bibliophile because I was drawn to books like some people are drawn to sweets—I couldn't get enough of them. And if I managed to get my hands on an especially captivating one, I would have to refrain from devouring it all in one sitting because I didn't want it to end.

The books on my nightstand in the summer of 1963 reflected my then taste in literature, e.g., *Catcher in the Rye, The Diary of a Young Girl, To Kill a Mockingbird*. When I got to high school, these and other acclaimed works often topped the required reading lists of my AP English courses. Some fifty-plus decades later, these and many comparable works of literature began dominating very different kinds of lists—compilations containing titles of books banned in schools and libraries throughout the US.

By then I was living in Florida, which was often neck and neck with Texas in the race to see which would win the annual distinction of being the state with the greatest number of banned book titles. The dubious honor went to Florida in 2022-23, motivating me to join the 451 Avengers, a South Florida grassroots organization. Its mission? To increase awareness of book banning and promote efforts to stop it. The name is a reference to Ray Bradbury's dystopian novel, *Fahrenheit 451* — the temperature at which paper burns.

I also joined a book club devoted to reading banned books where members took turns facilitating the monthly meetings. The week before my first time as moderator, I was literally brought to my knees by a GI bug that had me doing laps between my bedroom and bathroom. Determined not to let the group down, I kept my cell phone on my night table and my iPad on the bathroom sink counter and managed to finish Maia Kobabe's autobiographical graphic novel, *Gender Queer* and come up with suitable discussion prompts by the scheduled date.

But on that sultry summer night in 1963, when I was too tired to read even the lightweight fluff of a teen magazine, I knew whatever malady I had was more than just a stomach flu. I did manage to lift myself out of bed and use the bathroom again, but it didn't take a rocket scientist to know that urine the color of deep saffron and light clay-colored stools were not WNL (within normal limits). My suspicions were confirmed when Dr. Beecher came to see me after his office hours for the day were over. (Yes, some doctors still made house calls back then.) After my unpleasant visit to Evelyn's stepfather, my family had switched to using Dr. Beecher. He was decidedly jollier and with his white beard, mustache, and prominent paunch, bore an uncanny resemblance to Santa Claus.

When he finished examining me from head to toe, he solemnly stated that I needed to go to the hospital for some tests. He suspected that I had hepatitis A, an infectious disease caused by oral-fecal transmission. It's one of the pre-pandemic reasons why restrooms display signs warning their employees to wash hands thoroughly after using the facility.

I spent the next three weeks in the local hospital. By the time I was declared fit enough to start my sophomore year at James Madison High School, the semester was well underway and the cutoff for taking part in SING, the annual fall musical, had passed. When tickets went on sale for the November performances, I was one of the first in line. After seeing the talent and creativity displayed onstage by my peers, I vowed that come next November, I too would be a member of Madison's most popular extracurricular club.

* Pop quiz choices and their associated colors:
a) blue) b) reddish-purple c) cherry pink

Chapter 7

Sing Song

*Song: "Sing a Song" from **Sesame Street**, sung by The Carpenters*

"In brief, SING is a particular NY teenage phenomenon. Based on summer camp color-war competitions as well as varsity and variety shows, SING is a yearly student-run musical competition that pits grades against each other for best original show, and with awards granted in different categories. A signature of the SING show is the use of song parodies; students borrow the tune of a familiar song (from pop, rock 'n' roll, Broadway, folk, etc.) and write their own lyrics."

~ Ellen Levitt, Special to the
Brooklyn Daily Eagle, February 22, 2017.

My first experience with SING was during my sister's senior year at Abraham Lincoln HS in Coney Island. Unlike most school musicals, it is open to anyone who wants to be in it. Yes, there are auditions for lead and supporting roles but even if you can't carry a tune, you can be in the chorus where your off-key singing will be muted by as many as a hundred students surrounding you. In that era, New York City high schools contained upward of a thousand students per grade, so it was not unusual to have 10 percent or more of a given class taking part in SING.

My tone-deaf sister was a member of the chorus. My parents took me along to see her in it as they knew how much I loved musicals. From the minute the curtain went up I was mesmerized. I had never heard a song parody before. When the student orchestra struck up the opening to "Lullaby of Broadway" and the refrain morphed into "Lullaby of Lincoln," I was hooked. I couldn't get the tune out of my head.

Even today, whenever and wherever I hear the original show tune, I am transported back to that hard wooden auditorium seat watching Susan and her classmates having the time of their lives, already envisioning the day when I would get the opportunity to do likewise on the same stage.

By the time I was ready for high school, districts had been rezoned and Lincoln was no longer my neighborhood school. Luckily, there was a long SING tradition at Madison, so I was able to follow in my sister's footsteps. In addition to signing up for the junior year chorus, I joined the script committee. The school theme for that year was Broadway musicals by the Tony Award-winning team of Alan Jay Lerner and Frederick Loewe. The junior class was assigned the team's first big success, *Brigadoon*, which debuted in 1947. The plot revolves around two Americans who become lost while on a trip to Scotland. Eventually they find themselves in a mystical place called Brigadoon that doesn't appear on any maps and where the inhabitants seem to be living in a time warp.

Sound familiar? If so, you probably know about *Schmigadoon!*, the hysterically funny send-up cocreated by and costarring Cecily Strong of *Saturday Night Live*. I learned about the show while listening to her interview with National Public Radio's Terry Gross during my drive back from Bagelfest. When Terry mentioned she was a big fan of musicals while growing up in Brooklyn, I wondered if perhaps she had been a SING participant in her high school years. Sure enough, research revealed Terry had been on the script committee at Sheepshead Bay HS.

"So, I was one of the lyricists for each year that I was there. And part of the time I was in high school my friends shared this interest in theater, and it was great, and I thought, if I could live that life where there's theater and there's song and there's music and people designing scenery and painting it, that would just be super. And then I thought, how do you get there? How the hell do you get there? But it was kind of thrilling if somebody sang a lyric that I wrote. Like once I was walking down the street and I heard a couple of the basketball players singing a lyric that I wrote and I thought, that is really—that's just fabulous."

Like Terry, I gravitated to the creative rather than the performance side of SING although the ham in me would have loved to land a feature role. I did manage to make a brief appearance onstage in my senior year when I wrote and performed a comic number from Harnick and Bock's *Fiorello,* spoofing JFK's Presidential Fitness Test. Entering from the back doors of the auditorium dressed in my gym suit and sneakers, I ran down the center aisle singing my own words:

I'm physically unfit

I lack coordination

But for your benefit

I'll give a demonstration

I'll do my best

To try to pass the test:

Once onstage, I performed a series of poorly executed sit-ups, squat thrusts, and jumping jacks, earning a solid round of applause at the end.

Even though I was carrying a heavy academic load because I thought that I might want to go to medical school and SING took up a lot of my time, it was not the only activity I did at Madison. I wrote for the yearbook, assisted in the program office, served as Girl Leader of Arista, the school's honor society and was a twirler (as was Ruth Bader Ginsburg who, believe it or not, went by the nickname "Kiki" when she attended Madison). But SING was my favorite. Like Terry Gross, I was not exactly sure how to parlay my avocation into a career, but I did have a germ of an idea.

When it came time to meet with my guidance counselor, Mrs. Kalowitz, I strode into her office and confidently announced, "I want to go to an out-of-town school with a good musical theater program so that I can become a Broadway lyricist."

Mrs. K peered over her wire-rimmed glasses with a skeptical look and replied, "That's not a profession for a bright young Brooklyn girl like you.* With your GPA and science grades, better you should stick to your original career goal and become a doctor. Choose one of the city colleges or NY state universities, all of which have excellent premed programs. You can live at home and use your NYS Regents scholarship toward tuition. That'll save you lots of money that can then be used to help pay for medical school." She handed me the relevant applications, bid me farewell, and beckoned the next student on deck to come in.

That night at dinner, I told my parents and sister about the "guidance" I received earlier in the day. My mother and father were on board with Mrs. K's recommendations. And since they didn't want me going out of town, they felt Brooklyn College made the most sense. Susan grasped my disappointment and immediately went to bat for me.

"At least let her go to one of the out-of-town state schools. That way she can keep her NYS Regents scholarship, experience dorm life, and still be close enough to come home for weekends and vacations."

Bolstered by her support, I rummaged around the house for a NY state map to determine the location of the state school farthest from Brooklyn. Turned out to be Buffalo, the farthest I could go without leaving the US (a definite plus in my mind), but a city whose winter temperatures tended to vary from subzero to merely frigid. This sobering statistic was more than offset by the fact that the State University of NY at Buffalo (UB for short), was ranked highest in the constellation of NYS colleges and universities at that time. I announced, "Buffalo's the school for me." It was obvious my parents were not happy with my decision.

"It's really very far away," they moaned. Luckily, Susan came to my rescue once again. "Buffalo is one of the stops in Dad's sales territory. He can visit Joan during the several times a year that he travels on the road. (Translation: He would be able to check up on me periodically and report back to my mother.) So, I had Susan to thank for helping me make my first major life decision. Little did I know that some twelve years later she would guide me to make an even more life-changing one.

Carole King, Madison 1958, played piano for freshman SING. She went on to become an iconic female songwriter/singer with well more than a hundred hit singles, several of which compiled the score of the hit Broadway musical, Beautiful.

Chapter 8

Shuffle Off to Buffalo

Song: "Buffalo Gals" sung by Pete Seeger

O ne of my favorite songs, Dusty Springfield's "You Don't Have to Say You Love Me," reached number one on the pop charts the same year I started college. So, I took this as a positive omen when it came on the radio just as my parents and I turned off the New York State Thruway at the exit for Buffalo. It served as an affirmation that I was right to make the University of Buffalo my first choice when deciding where to spend my college years.

My mother, on the other hand, began to have some doubts when we arrived at my assigned room in Clement Hall, one of two freshman dorms. My roommate had preceded our arrival, as was apparent from the crucifix prominently displayed over the neatly made bed and the rosary beads curled up on the chest of drawers next to it.

"Vey iz mir," she intoned as if these trappings signified I would be living with a religious zealot who would try to convert me to Catholicism by the time Rosh Hashanah rolled around. In her defense, there had been a brief period in my life when I lamented my Jewish heritage and wished I had been born a Catholic. Granted, I was about seven at the time—the age when young Christian girls don white, frilly, fairy-tale-like frocks with matching veils and white gloves to take their First Communion. I was entranced by the sight of these miniature brides preening as they posed for photos in front of the neighborhood houses, surrounded by equally beaming family members. The fanciest dress in my wardrobe back then was a modest navy number more suitable for funerals than weddings. I beseeched my mother to buy me one of these child bride's dresses.

"Only shiksas get to wear those outfits," she disdainfully told me.

"What's a shiksa?"

"Girls who aren't Jewish—like your Catholic friend, Maria."

"You mean Maria Passalacqua? She can't be Catholic. I think her family is from an Indian tribe. You know, like Minnehaha."

Our second-grade class had just finished a unit on American Indians (this was around 1957, decades before the term "Native Americans" came into usage.) Our teacher, Mrs. Garbow, taught us Minnehaha was a Dakota word for waterfall or rapid water but was often translated to mean "laughing water," probably because of the gurgling sound made by water tumbling over rocks. And that a famous author named Henry Wadsworth Longfellow had given that name to a fictional character in a famous poem called "The Song of Hiawatha" that begins with the oft-quoted line, "On the shores of Gitche Gumee."

With the similarity in cadence between both four-syllable names and the two long black braids that fell to her waist, my seven-year-old brain free-associated that Maria was an Indian girl, just like Hawthorne's heroine. My mother proceeded to give me an Ancestry.com-lite explanation for my confusion.

"Maria's parents were born in Italy. Sicily, I think. Sicilians are usually darker skinned than Italians from other parts of Italy. That's why she has such beautiful black hair. Her family attends St. Edmund's Church over on Avenue T and Ocean Avenue."

And that's when I think I had my very first "aha" moment. Of course, Maria wasn't Indian. She was one of several students who took part in a "released time" program that allowed students to be excused from school an hour earlier every Wednesday to study the Confraternity of Christian Doctrine (CCD), more commonly referred to as catechism. Those of us left behind were green with envy at this educational equivalent of the prized "Get Out of Jail Free" card that we prayed for when we played Monopoly. Ten years later when I was assigned a blond-haired, blue-eyed Irish lass from upstate New York as my freshman roommate and learned more about her religious upbringing, I realized my early childhood desire to convert just so I could look like a child bride would not have been a good trade-off because I most definitely would have wound up a lapsed Catholic.

Pat Donnelly, on the other hand, was the exact opposite. A Syracuse, NY native, she had gone to parochial school all her life, attended mass every Sunday, and during freshman orientation, she joined Newman Club, the Catholic equivalent of Hillel. Yet we were very much alike in other ways. We were very organized so our room was never a slovenly mess like most of the others on our floor, we both were elected to Freshman Class Council during orientation and we each entered UB planning to pursue health care careers—she in pharmacy. As a result, our course loads were almost identical. Which turned out to be very helpful when a second medicinal lemon landed in my lap before the semester even began. (Sound familiar?)

Instead of spending my first day in a classroom, I was confined to bed. Earlier in the week I had begun to experience minor discomfort every time I swallowed. When it got worse, I figured I'd better check in with the infirmary for a quick strep test as a precaution, and I tested positive. I did not anticipate I wouldn't be allowed to check out the same day. I ended up staying five days, missing two calculus classes, three inorganic chemistry lectures, and a lab.

I called Pat and asked if she could bring me the homework assignments as well as copies of her notes. (Thanks to the nuns in her elementary school, she had perfect penmanship so I knew they would be legible.) No sooner had I hung up the phone than she showed up at the door to the infirmary. I was so relieved I wanted to give her a huge hug, but visitors weren't allowed inside. So, I blew her a kiss as she handed over the materials I'd requested. To this day, I'm convinced I wouldn't have gotten an A in those courses had it not been for Pat.

Pat and I had two wonderful suitemates—Louise and Sharon. They were also taking science prerequisites for health care majors: Louise wanted to be a nurse and Sharon, a physical therapist. Like Pat, both hailed from small towns in upstate New York. The fact that I was the only one of the four who grew up "downstate" was not a coincidence. Out of my high school graduating class of 1,216, a large percentage chose to attend UB, including Evelyn, my best friend from fourth grade and Rob, my senior-year boyfriend. Since the whole appeal of going out of town for college was to broaden my horizons and meet people from different backgrounds than the ones who had "peopled" my life for the past seventeen years, I specified a preference for a roommate who was not from the NYC metropolitan area when I had filled out the housing request form over the summer.

The four of us turned out to be remarkably compatible, although they were fond of teasing me about my Brooklyn accent. The first time it happened was about two weeks into the semester, when we deliberated whether to eat someplace other than the cafeteria for a change. "Here's my idea," I proposed. "Let's go to dinner in the student union." Only *idea* came out sounding like *idear* and *dinner* as *dinna*. The three of them rolled their eyes and laughed. Pat finally spoke up. "Joan, if you remove the *R* from *idea* and put it at the end of *dinna*, you've got a deal." I retaliated by saying, "OK, Pee-at," imitating the flat *A* pronunciation of her name. But no matter how hard I concentrated, I never did get the hang of this linguistic correction or, for that matter, saying "Long Island" instead of *Long Guy Land,* another hallmark of Brooklynese.

As the term wore on, I met a lot of other students and began to spend less time with my dorm posse. In French class, I became friendly with Bonnie Becker, whose light eyes, fair skin, and straight blond bob give her the appearance of a Dutch maiden from Amsterdam. In fact, she was of Ashkenazic ancestry, born and raised in Baldwin, a suburb on Long Island. And her mother grew up in Brooklyn and went to my high school. What were the odds of that?

Bonnie lived in Goodyear Hall, the other freshman dorm. Through her I met two more Goodyear residents: Jackie Moss and Ellen Seigel. They soon became my new posse and together we went to fraternity parties, football games, Hillel holiday dinners, and concerts on and off campus.

When it came time to declare a choice for sophomore year roommates, Bonnie and I signed up as a pair; Jackie and Ellen did likewise. We asked to live in Macdonald Hall, a small dorm with a kitchen in the basement so we wouldn't have to rely on the university's meal plan. And it was closer to the academic buildings on campus so we wouldn't have as far to walk to classes, an important variable given Buffalo's "white winters" and gusty winds. These were just some of the changes that were in store for us as we headed into sophomore year.

Chapter 9

Permit Me to Digress

Song: "The Times They Are a-Changin'" sung by Bob Dylan

Speaking of changes, I think you should know something about me. I am an analog person living in a digital world. When it comes to fully understanding how computers, smartphones, and remote-control devices operate, I am technologically challenged. Which is kind of ironic because in my sophomore year of college, I eagerly enrolled in one of the first computer programming courses to be offered at UB. It was taught by a professor named Anthony Ralston who seemed rather jolly for a techie type. He cheerfully taught Fortran, the name of the decidedly "uncheerful" program we were expected to master. He might as well have been speaking Urdu as far as I was concerned, since most of what he said went right over my head.

With the help of my classmates, I eventually managed to operationalize his instructions and produce an elementary program. However, it was a very labor-intensive process that involved keypunching instructions on beige cards using something called a CRT machine (damned if I can remember what the acronym stood for), then feeding them into the computer. Mind you, this was in the era before personal computers were developed. The only way to accomplish this tedious task was to trek over to the university computer center, wait until a mainframe machine became available, input the cards, and trek back the next morning to retrieve them along with the reams of computer paper that hopefully displayed the printed counterpart of what had been extrapolated from the keypunched holes.

Needless to say, I did not enroll in the second semester of the course because I preferred spending my evenings engaged in more enjoyable pastimes such as trekking off campus to the Beef and Ale House, a local hangout on Main Street. Its specialty was a Western New York staple and remains the most delicious sandwich I've ever had in my life: beef on weck, shorthand for thinly sliced rare roast beef au jus covered with horseradish and served on kummelweck, a crusty kaiser roll sprinkled with coarse salt and caraway seeds rather than the customary poppy seed topping. Try my best, I've never managed to find another roast beef sandwich that quite measures up to it.

Despite being a Fortran flunk-out, I did manage to acquire the ABCs of surviving in a virtual world—emailing, Googling, and texting. I'm pretty proficient in the first two but lag behind in the third. It always amazes me how fast most people reply to my texts because it takes me what seems like an eternity to type them. My rather wide fingers are not as nimble as I'd like them to be in composing a message on the tiny spaces that pass for a keyboard on my iPhone. I have had to resort to the pecking-with-one-finger method and harbor insane jealousy of preteens who text with the alacrity of a concert pianist playing "Flight of the Bumblebee." To compound the problem, my husband couldn't stand the sound of that high-pitched little *ding* that pings whenever a text message arrives. Why is it he is able to hear the sound of this new age gizmo when he's two rooms away yet totally unresponsive to the decades-old Winchester Cathedral ringtone of our front doorbell that's loud enough to summon parishioners to church from two towns over? He demanded that I disable it; I complied. This wasn't a battle worth fighting.

That is why the only way I know someone has texted me is when I check my phone, which isn't very often. This apparently enrages my hyperactive friends who turn all huffy when more than a nanosecond goes by before they hear from me. "Why didn't you answer my text sooner? We were looking for a sub for our mahjongg game…a week from Friday." This brings me to the other reason why they don't get an instantaneous reply. I've implemented a triage system for the order in which I respond to texts or return phone calls. It's simple, really; if they don't include the words *blood, fire, flood* or the numerals *9-1-1*, they default to a mental queue in descending order of priority.

I haven't succumbed to the new age allure of a Kindle or Nook either. I prefer the tactile sensation of turning pages and dog-earing them so weeks or even years later, I can easily go back and find the lines of inspirational prose or stanzas of poetry I thought would remain forever emblazoned in my brain, so profound they seemed upon the first run-through.

There's also a sense of nostalgia attached to the pre-online method of reading because it transports me back in time to my childhood, much of which was spent huddled under the covers in my pink wallpapered bedroom, a comic book, magazine, or novel in my hands. Seeing additional reading material piled high on the night table next to me gave me a visual reminder that more

pleasure was in store immediately after finishing whatever printed material was capturing my attention at that very moment. Plus,
practically speaking, if I happened to fall asleep with a book on my
chest, I didn't have to worry that it would shatter into shards of
broken glass and plastic and cost a small fortune to replace if I were
to roll over and knock it to the floor. The worst that could happen?
I might lose my place.

On the other hand, I was an early adaptor of word processing
thanks to my seventh grade typing teacher, Mrs. Hirsch; otherwise,
you wouldn't be reading this book because I don't have the pa-
tience to write in longhand. Nevertheless, I am constantly ridiculed
for still using Microsoft Word because almost everyone who's anyone has switched to Google Documents.

But when it comes to social media, don't even get me started. When I first heard about "influencers going viral," I thought
it was a tongue-in-cheek reference to an increase in the spread of
different strains of seasonal "influenzas." Of course, this was back
when corona was simply the name of a beer not the designation of
a deadly pathogen. As for Reddit, Pinterest, and Twitter (as the site
was known before Elon Musk downsized it to a single letter of the
alphabet), they could be partners in a high-profile, white-shoe law
firm for all I know.

Confession: I did break down and join Facebook after the
birth of my granddaughter Marissa because I suspected I would
never see photos of her or her brother if I didn't. Over the years
I've managed to learn how to utilize some of its other features and
was beginning to feel somewhat proud of my prowess until just
recently. Said granddaughter—at the age of eleven—overheard me
talking to her mother about an interesting FB posting sent by a mutual friend. She turned to me with a look of utter disdain and chid-

ed, "Nonny, Facebook is for old people. You have to get on Insta. Give me your phone." Reluctantly, I complied. "And TikTok too. So you can see all the videos I've made. My last one blew up. I have over a hundred followers. Let me show you."

So, you can certainly understand why a Luddite like me was filled with apprehension when I realized I would have to master yet another internet curveball as the world headed into lockdown in March 2020. Until then, I'd only heard the word *zoom* used as a verb or an adjective, as in "zoom around town" or "use a zoom shot in the next scene." As my grandchildren know, I am a stickler for correct word usage. My reputation has earned me the designation of "the grammar police." Their worst transgressions involve pronouns: "Me and Jesse want to go to the mall." Ugh! The sound of it grates on my ears as jarringly as chalk squeaking on a blackboard. I refrain from telling them that because I know they will have a caustic comeback. "Get real, Nonny. Blackboards are so yesterday. We use whiteboards in school nowadays."

As we all now know, "in school" took on a whole new meaning once COVID-19 began ruling our lives. Students were able to go to class without ever leaving their homes or getting out of their pajamas, thanks to virtual learning platforms such as Zoom. And they could interact with their friends and relatives in real time despite the confinement of quarantine thanks to Zoom's conference-style capabilities. Which is how I came to embrace this verb/adjective turned noun. With the help of my IT guy—my grandson Ryan—I downloaded the app and used it to throw a virtual party to celebrate Larry's and my golden wedding anniversary, fifty years to the day that we married, Sunday, June 14, 1970.

I had to spring for the extra cost of hosting more people than the free Zoom app allowed because my guest list was so large. It included people from as far back as elementary school to new neighbors who had moved to my condo community just a few months before. And of course, my friends from UB who are scattered across the US: Bonnie and another friend, Judy, live in California; Ellen divides her time between Naples, Florida and Rochester, New York and Jackie lives not far from where she grew up on Long Island. My senior year roommate, a high school classmate also named Joan, resides in Rhode Island.

Because of these geographical constraints, we have rarely been able to gather together in person. After seeing the technological success of my Zoom party, Ellen suggested that we try holding regularly scheduled virtual get-togethers on Zoom and Jackie agreed to be the host. Ever since, we've been convening as "The Buffalo Gals" on the third Wednesday of every month. Inevitably we end up reminiscing about our college years all of which took place against the backdrop of the Vietnam War, an epic period that irrevocably changed the course of so many lives. In fact, had it not been for the change in the cultural climate of campus life wrought by the protest movement of the late sixties, my life might have taken a very different turn.

Chapter 10

Where the Boys Are

Song: "Where the Boys Are" sung by Connie Francis

The first change I encountered when I returned to UB in the fall of 1967 was a welcome one—a revision to the dress code. Up until then, women were not allowed to wear pants in the dining halls, an arbitrary sartorial sanction in keeping with the cultural mores of the time but one that didn't make much sense given Buffalo's weather conditions. Fall foliage season was short-lived and trudging through snow to take final exams in May was not considered a freakish phenomenon. The city's location on the shores of Lake Erie exponentially worsened the situation due to what was known as the lake effect.

Since all first-year female students were housed in either Goodyear or Clement Hall, both of which connected through interior passageways to a shared dining hall, I never had to brave the elements for any of my meals during freshman year. In Macdonald Hall we were assigned to use the dining facilities housed in a nearby freestanding building, Tower Hall—the only all-male dormitory on campus. Traversing the short distance from one dorm to the other was a breeze—literally speaking. The breeze turned into a tornado when the wind whipped off Lake Erie, creating a wind tunnel between the two resident halls.

Coupled with the frigid temperatures and snowstorms that prevailed throughout most of the academic year, this made the two-minute walk seem like an eternity unless you were wearing thick woolen pants over heavy tights while doing it. Luckily, my friends and I were spared this ordeal thanks to the elimination of the discriminatory clause in the university's dress code, although we did miss the Clement benefit of not having to go outside at all. (We still had that option since we could just hunker down in the basement kitchen of Macdonald and prepare our own meals assuming we had remembered to lay in supplies in advance.)

In freshman year, I had signed up for skiing to fulfill my gym requirement and at the start of sophomore year, I joined Schussmeisters, the UB ski club, as did Bonnie, Judy, Ellen, and Jackie. The club met every Tuesday night at Kissing Bridge, a ski area about an hour away. Bus transportation was included in the dues, which increased our chances for socializing with students who lived off campus.

And socialize I did. In fact, I was having such a good time that my priorities shifted from academics to activities. Instead of the required premed requisites of Organic Chemistry and Biology, I opted for Art History and Music History so I would be better able to appreciate the offerings at Buffalo's cultural institutions such as the Albright Knox Museum, Studio Arena Theatre, and Kleinhans Music Hall. The concerts at Kleinhans whetted my appetite for classical music and I began listening to WBFO, the campus radio station. It was housed in Baird Hall, not far from Macdonald, and aired a weekly program featuring well-known compositions from the traditional canon. The opening theme music was the sprightly first movement of Mendelssohn's Italian Symphony, conjuring up images of signors and signoras dressed in the latest Milan fashions sipping limoncello in the gardens of Tuscan villas.

After a few bars, the soothing voice of the program host was heard as the music faded out. "Hello, I'm Thomas Clark. Welcome to the *Classical Hour* here at WBFO." For the next sixty minutes, I listened spellbound as he deejayed one beautiful composition after another. One blustery afternoon, on a whim I decided to walk over to Baird while he was on the air, hoping to catch him afterward. The station was housed in two small rooms on the second floor, each about the size of a closet, connected by a tiny vestibule. There was a guy in each of them, both seated behind mikes and wearing headphones. I rightly surmised the disheveled one with the long, stringy hair, scrawny beard, and Grateful Dead T-shirt was the studio engineer and the on-air personality was the clean-cut fellow wearing pressed corduroys and a tweed sports coat with leather elbow patches, pipe protruding from the breast pocket.

I positioned myself in full view of the latter, smiled coyly, and patiently waited until he signed off the air. I then confided that I was a regular listener and wanted to meet the man with the mellifluous voice. Flattered, he offered to give me a tour of the station, which took all of about a minute. There was nothing much to see other than a desk, water cooler, and next to it, a waist-high machine resembling a typewriter from which staccato clicking noises emanated intermittently. The attention-getting sound was vaguely familiar; eventually it dawned on me that I'd heard it many times before in newsreels as well as movies and TV shows set in newsrooms.

The source was a teletype machine that conveyed news stories from wire services such as Associated Press (AP) and United Press International (UPI) to broadcast stations and newspapers. Tom looked at me mesmerized by the reams of paper that the machine was spewing out. He ripped off a sheet containing a local news story and handed it to me. While the content was not earth-shattering, the mere fact that I was likely to learn about an event before anyone else tuning in to that evening's newscast would, provided a kind of smug satisfaction. I mustered up the gumption to tell Tom I'd like to volunteer as a WBFO newscaster. He grinned knowingly and handed me a business card.

"Call Henry Tenenbaum. He's the station manager and does all the hiring. Keep in mind, he won't start you off in a prime-time spot and you will have to be on call to sub when someone calls in sick or more likely hungover."

"That's OK. My course load is much lighter this year since I dropped premed courses. And I live on campus, so I don't have to worry about getting stuck in traffic or driving through a blizzard."

"Great. Let me know how it goes with Henry. Come on, I'll walk out with you."

And that marked the start of my relationship with WBFO as well as Tom. He was a "townie" with an undergraduate degree from Cornell, enrolled in UB's graduate program in biochemistry. Our social life revolved around potluck parties at the homes of his fellow grad students, most of who were married with children. In December, he invited me to participate in his family's traditional Yuletide ritual: watching *How The Grinch Stole Christmas* while sipping eggnog and eating his mother's kuchenbuchen, a baked good that made two-week-old fruitcake taste like tarte aux pommes. And so began the decline of my relationship with Tom.

Seeing him in the bosom of his close-knit Irish Catholic family as they sat around a gloriously bedecked Christmas tree in the living room of their Victorian house, I realized that a long-term relationship with him wasn't in the cards. Our backgrounds were just too different for it to have worked. By the time the New Year's Eve confetti had been cleared from Times Square, I already had a successor in sight.

Ezra was also a townie, but his parents were Holocaust survivors and he lacked Tom's Ivy League pedigree. He commuted to UB as an undergraduate, leaving after three years to enroll in its dental school. I met him when Bonnie began dating his friend, Mark. Ezra's boyish good looks and shy smile captured my attention, so I convinced Bonnie to have Mark introduce us. I was thrilled when he asked me out then crestfallen when ten days went by after our initial date without a peep from him. My spirits rose when he finally called and asked me out for the coming Saturday, only to be dashed when the same post-date pattern happened again. This "wax on, wax off" routine was straight out of Mr. Miyagi's playbook in *The Karate Kid* and it drove me crazy. When I found out that dental school remained in session during the time I was scheduled to go home for midwinter intersession, I hatched a Machiavellian scheme designed to convince Ezra I was worthy of more attention than he'd been paying me.

I told my parents I wouldn't be coming home for Washington's birthday weekend because I had signed up to take part in an extracurricular psych experiment. In fact, I did plan on engaging in a research study of sorts—investigating the whereabouts of Ezra while he was on campus without having my classes, homework, or WBFO shifts to take up my time in hopes I would casually run into him, strike up a conversation, and entice him to come to my dorm room for some 'R and R' after he'd finished studying. Or to put it another way—I planned on stalking him. (Don't look so shocked—I owned up to my stalker instincts a few chapters back.)

Spoiler alert: Not a single sighting of him despite hours hanging out in the dental school library, cafeteria, or the student union. It wasn't until a year later that I discovered he had a serious girlfriend all along who lived in Buffalo but went to Buffalo State Teachers College and that I wasn't the only UB coed in his rotation schedule.

Thankfully, I didn't spend too much time lamenting my failed espionage attempt because Bonnie, Jackie, and Ellen convinced me to accompany them to Miami Beach on spring break. We booked two adjacent rooms in the oceanfront Thunderbird Hotel on Collins Avenue and 184th Street. A few blocks away was Rascal House, a Jewish deli known for the baskets of mouthwatering Danish, rolls, and other baked goods that sat side by side heaping bowls of pickles and sauerkraut, all of which were free with your meal. It quickly became our go-to breakfast hangout. We ordered the cheapest menu items then surreptitiously squirreled the complimentary goodies in our pocketbooks, the better to nosh on later in the day at poolside.

There, we slathered ourselves in baby oil and stretched out on what passed for chaise lounges at our modest lodgings, in pursuit of a golden tan designed to make our friends green with envy when we returned to campus. Instead, we got second-degree sunburns. To assuage our discomfort, we headed to Jahn's Ice Cream Parlor, home of the Kitchen Sink Sundae—a gargantuan confection consisting of gobs of ice cream smothered in boatloads of whipped cream and syrup that the management refuses to serve to less than eight people.

No one in our group was much of a drinker so our social life was on the staid side. At night we would grab a bite to eat and *shpatzir* (Yiddish for stroll) along the strip of motels up and down

Collins Avenue. One evening we had dinner at a noisy pub. We had to strain to hear each other because a TV was mounted to the wall right across from our table and the bar was crowded with customers shouting to be heard over one another. Suddenly, an agitated voice cried out: "Pipe down and turn up the TV." A hush descended as the bartender extended his arm to comply.

"We interrupt this broadcast to bring you breaking news. Stay tuned for details."

Chapter 11

Shot Down Again…and Again

Song: "Abraham, Martin and John" sung by Dion

April 4, 1968

"**G**ood evening. **Dr. Martin Luther King Jr.**, the apostle of nonviolence in the civil rights movement, has been shot to death in Memphis, TN. Dr. King was standing on the balcony of a second-floor hotel room as the shot was fired from across the street."

Stunned, the four of us sat transfixed as Walter Cronkite of *CBS News* announced the assassination of the visionary leader and social activist. The replay of the footage from the balcony was followed by reports of incipient rioting taking place throughout the country. Eventually we uprooted ourselves from the table and walked back to our hotel. Just a few days of spring break remained but the fun of frolicking on the beach had washed out. On the somber flight back to Buffalo, I found myself thinking about the day JFK died. I was a sophomore in high school at the time.

November 22, 1963. I was just about to take my seat in Mrs. Glaubiger's geometry class when someone ran by in the hall, shouting, "Have you heard? President Kennedy's been shot." I jumped to my feet in disbelief as chaos broke out. After what seemed like an eternity but in reality was probably just thirty minutes, an announcement emanated from the overhead speaker declaring his death had been confirmed by Walter Cronkite at approximately 1:38 p.m. As I walked home in shock that afternoon, I couldn't help but think we'd have little to be thankful for, come Thanksgiving the following Thursday in the wake of such sadness.

Five years later, I and the rest of the country had barely recovered from the loss of JFK when we were confronted with another American tragedy.

June 5, 1968. Robert F. Kennedy was celebrating his victory in the California Democratic presidential primary at the Ambassador Hotel in Los Angeles when he was fatally shot by Sirhan Sirhan. Two months earlier, he had been campaigning in Indianapolis where he was scheduled to make a stop in a predominantly African American neighborhood on the night MLK Jr. was assassinated. Fearful that violence might break out and endanger his safety, many of his staff members urged him to cancel his appearance. Instead, he proceeded to calmly address the crowd, advising them "what we need in the United States is not hatred; what we need in the United States is not violence and lawlessness, but is love, and wisdom and compassion toward one another...to tame the savageness of man and make gentle the life of this world."

I was home alone when I heard that RFK had been assassinated. Without the benefit of family, high school friends, or college dorm mates to share my sorrow and grief, I was at loose ends. As hard as I tried, I couldn't fall asleep that night. Maybe it's because I sensed that this latest senseless murder of a revered world-renowned icon wouldn't be the last in my lifetime.

December 8, 1980. Another sleepless night. Second year of med school. I was downing cups of caffeinated coffee in order to cram for the microbiology exam scheduled for the next day—December 9. It was not until I arrived on campus that I heard the devastating news—John Lennon had been murdered outside the entrance to his Central Park West apartment building the night before. His killer? A disaffected young man named Mark David Chapman. Chapman, born in 1955, was a fan of J.D. Salinger's *The Catcher in the Rye.* He identified with its protagonist, Holden Caulfield, who cannot abide all the "phonies" he meets. In Chapman's mind, Lennon was a hypocrite because his admonition to "imagine no possessions" belied his lavish lifestyle. Lennon needed to be killed. Too bad Chapman was inspired by the prose of Salinger's fiction rather than the poetry of RFK's speech but then again, he was only thirteen years old on that fateful night in Memphis in 1968.

I had just turned nineteen at the time of King's murder and was almost halfway through college. Spring break 1968 turned out to be more somber than celebratory, so when I heard that the UB Ski Club was planning a trip to Innsbruck, Austria at the conclusion of the fall 1968 semester, I eagerly signed up despite its steep price tag. The next step would be to convince my parents to let me go. I figured if I got a job right away, I could save up enough money by Christmas, providing me with a sound argument to overcome parental resistance. Thus, in addition to carrying a full course load and putting in my allotted hours at WBFO, I took a part-time job.

I was lucky to secure a coveted position working at Norton Hall, the Student Union, located squarely in the middle of campus. My job fell under the heading of hospitality management. The building housed a cafeteria, bowling alley, rathskeller, two meeting rooms for movies, lectures, and shows, and two student lounges.

Over the years, each lounge had come to have its own identity. Commuting students tended to congregate in The Dorothy Hass Lounge, named after a former dean of student affairs. But no one ever called it that. It was universally referred to as the "townie lounge." Fraternity members hung out in a smaller space dubbed "the animal lounge," nestled between the coat check room and the campus newsstand.

Even though copies of the *Buffalo Evening News* and the *Toronto Globe* and *Mail* coupled with packages of Marlboros and Gauloises cigarettes (the preferred brand of Canadian members of the UB community) took up more space combined than the boxes of Milky Ways, Butterfingers, and Almond Joys, the shoebox-sized newsstand was affectionately referred to as the Norton candy stand. Depending on the weekly staffing roster, I floated between there and the much larger coat check room, which turned out to be one of the fringe benefits of the job. Since anyone walking from one end of campus to the other had to pass through Norton Hall, my vantage point from either location enabled me to familiarize myself with the comings and goings of passersby.

This proved quite useful for someone with serial stalking instincts such as *moi*. Whether I wanted to lobby for a grade change from a faculty member who refused to hold office hours (or one who did but was notorious for hitting on females), shake down reimbursement for all the tabs that I had picked up for penny-pinching friends whose excuse was always, "I only have big bills on hand" (I was always able to make change from the cash register), or catch the eye of that cute bookish guy three rows in front of me in statistics (who was a whiz in math), my job provided the necessary access to accomplish these tasks.

Unfortunately, there was a hefty downside when I was assigned to the candy stand—proximity to the candy. Whoppers were (and still are) my confectionary Achilles' heel. There was something almost orgasmic about that little burst of malted milk that erupted in my mouth when I bit into one. I tried to limit my craven caloric debauchery to one box a week, mitigating my guilt by assuming the manager of the student union had accounted for employee pilferage in the budget. I guess I was lucky I was not a smoker, or I probably would have wound up with a serious addiction to nicotine.

By the time I was ready to return home for Thanksgiving, I had accumulated a nice little nest egg. Counting on the likely possibility that my parents would be close to a serotonin-induced stupor after ingesting mounds of turkey and stuffing at one sitting, I decided to announce my plans for winter break just before dessert, hoping they would be too mellow to shoot them down.

"Absolutely not," my father bellowed. My mother agitatedly shook her head from side to side, uttering *"gottenyu"* under her breath.

"But the Ski Club got a great package deal on airfare and hotel. And I've saved up lots from my job, so you won't need to give me tons of money. In fact, the whole trip will cost you less than when I went to Miami Beach for spring break."

"It's not a matter of money," he went on.

"Then what is it exactly?"

"There's no way in hell any child of mine is going to vacation in Hitler's birthplace."

Damn! I never saw that coming. Mission aborted. They shot down my hopes. Knowing there was nothing I could have said or done to change their minds, I conceded defeat and surrendered to the urge to devour two slices of apple pie. No need for portion control. I wouldn't have to worry about squeezing into my already too small, size 14 ski pants come January 1969.

Chapter 12

Fly Me to the Moon

Song: "Fly Me to the Moon" sung by Frank Sinatra

Three weeks later I was back in Brooklyn. Felt as if I'd never left. The only difference? The holiday food on the table. Brisket had replaced turkey; potato latkes substituted for stuffing; and rugelach appeared at the end of the meal instead of apple pie. It was Hanukkah, 1968. At that time, it was still considered a minor Jewish holiday celebrating the Maccabean revolt against King Antiochus.

You would have been hard-pressed to find any Hanukkah sentiments on Hallmark cards at the corner drugstore (this was way before Rite Aid and CVS drove out the small neighborhood pharmacies but that's a tale for another time), let alone giant menorahs perched alongside towering Christmas trees on the lawns of local municipal buildings. It hadn't yet morphed into the gift-giving extravaganza created to compete with the razzle-dazzle of Christmas, a day devoted to commemorating the birth of a nice Jewish boy who grew up to be a long-haired, sandal-wearing man whose mom thought he walked on water and whose dad was a father in name only. (Let's face it—how many statues of Joseph have you seen in museums?)

As the years went by, Jewish parents struggled to keep up with their gentile counterparts by emphasizing that Hannukah "outshone" Christmas—literally as well as numerically. By capitalizing on the fact it was a Festival of Lights that lasted not one but eight days, they came up with the rationale that their children were entitled to receive at least one present per day. We're not talking just token gifts, like a pair of Hello Kitty socks or a toy Matchbox car. High ticket and/or sought-after items were asked for and expected. Remember the Cabbage Patch Kids craze? Beanie Babies? Rushing like crazy to get to Toys "R" Us after work, praying you wouldn't come home empty-handed? Then thanks to Jeff Bezos, Amazon came along and helped level the playing field somewhat with its revolutionary online business model, making holiday shopping easier for parents of all denominations.

Then wouldn't you know it, some wise man (pun intended) came up with the idea of Elf on a Shelf, leaving Jewish *emas* and *abbas* (mothers and fathers) at a major disadvantage. How could they compete with such a clever idea? One Jewish dad married to a non-Jewish woman came to the rescue. A successful executive in the children's toy industry, Neal Hoffman, fought back by developing a similar product and coined an equally poetic name: Mensch on a Bench.

But the only trappings of Hanukkah to be found in the Rubenfeld residence circa 1968 were a plastic dreidel, an ashtray filled with a handful of chocolate gelt, and an electric menorah on the windowsill in the living room. My one present? A ten-dollar gift certificate to A&S, my mother's favorite Brooklyn department store, founded by two entrepreneurial members of the tribe: Abraham and Straus. If she and my father had not pulled the plug on the Innsbruck trip, I would have happily used it toward a new ski parka. But I was too bummed-out by the realization I was back in Brooklyn again to make the two-hour, round-trip subway trek to cash it in. Instead, I stuck it in my underwear drawer and sulked around the house until it was time to return to school to take my final exams.

I was booked on an early morning American Airlines flight to Buffalo out of LaGuardia Airport on the first Wednesday in January. I was flying on a special discount in effect for college students that allowed for half fare tickets if you went standby. When I got to the lounge at the boarding gate, it was already quite crowded so my chances of making it on that flight were not looking good. As I walked through the area searching for somewhere to sit, a very handsome man wearing a double-breasted glen plaid suit and reading a newspaper briefly diverted my attention. I finally managed to find a seat on the other side of the lounge, pulled out my English lit textbook, and settled in to study.

"Flight 278 to Buffalo will now begin boarding," came the announcement over the intercom. "Families traveling with small children and infants, passengers with special needs, and/or priority boarding passes are invited to board first." The fellow in the glen plaid suit stood up and joined the initial boarding group. Hmm. He was traveling alone, devoid of any obvious physical handicaps and didn't appear in need of any special TLC so why was he getting preferential treatment? Probably best to steer clear of him.

General boarding took quite a while but finally all passengers traveling on standby were summoned to the check-in counter. Dragging my carry-on bag behind me. I walked past row after row of filled seats until I finally spotted a vacant one between two men. I shoved my bag into the overhead compartment, climbed over the long legs of the one on the aisle and strapped myself into the middle seat. The one in the window seat had his head buried in *The Wall Street Journal* so I tried striking up a conversation with the other one. Turned out he was German.

After my halting attempts to retrieve some basic conversational phrases from German 101, I gave up and resumed reading my textbook. As the plane taxied down the runway, the window seat inhabitant folded up his paper, revealing him to be the man of mystery from the boarding lounge. Our eyes met giving our lips permission to speak. His name was Larry Liman, his Army Reserve membership entitled him to early boarding privileges and he worked for his family's jewelry business in Manhattan's diamond district. Ca-ching! Upon hearing this last piece of information, I was sufficiently intrigued to close my textbook, shove it into the pocket on the back of the seat in front of me, and coquettishly shift in my seat to give him my undivided attention.

For the next fifty minutes, we played a spirited game of Jewish geography. He was a Syracuse U. grad from Queens, knew Phil Diener, a family friend who had been my parents' go-to source for diamond jewelry over the course of their marriage, had a younger cousin Frank, a year ahead of me at UB, and an older married cousin Albert, who lived in a Buffalo suburb close to the campus. Albert was indirectly responsible for Larry's trip to Buffalo that day. Like many male college graduates in the late sixties, Larry had been worried about being drafted. Joining the Army Reserves was a much sought-after option but living in NYC meant there was enormous competition to gain a spot. Albert thought Reserve units in western NY might have more openings. He and his wife, Sandra, had suggested Larry stay with them while searching for a unit that would take him.

Luckily, the commander of a unit in nearby Batavia was Jewish. When he saw the religion engraved on Larry's dog tags was Hebrew, he welcomed him with open arms, which increased the Jewish population of the unit to two. Reservists had to first go through basic training, which Larry did at Fort Dix, New Jersey. After that, his commitment required him to spend one weekend a month with his unit in Batavia. That's where he was headed when he boarded the flight to Buffalo with me.

As we prepared for landing, he offered to drive me back to campus in the car he'd rented for his one-hour trip to Batavia. Of course, I accepted. Once the plane was on the tarmac and passengers started to disembark, a fellow classmate spotted me retrieving my luggage and asked if I wanted to share a ride back to campus. When I informed her of Larry's offer, she asked me to ask him if he wouldn't mind taking her as well. Ooh, tough call. I wanted to continue to monopolize his attention on the short ride from the airport. But at that point in my life, I had not yet mastered the art of saying no. I obliged. Of course, clueless Larry was unaware of my ulterior motive.

"No problem." And so our ménage à trois proceeded off the plane and into the car Larry had rented.

After dropping her off at her dorm, I directed him to Macdonald Hall. My heart skipped a beat when he asked for my phone number and wanted to know when I would be returning home. "Ten days from now, after my last final." He carried my bag to the front door and the last words he said were, "I will call when you get back."

I climbed the stairs to my second-floor dorm room, where Judy, Ellen, Bonnie, and Jackie were waiting for me, a wide smile spread from ear to ear on each of their faces.

"Oh my God," exclaimed Judy excitedly. "We happened to all be here and saw you get out of the car. Tell us everything."

Ten days later, I was just sitting down to dinner with my mother and sister when the phone rang. My mother got up to answer it. "It's for you, Joanie. Someone named Larry Liman?"

I practically leaped out of my chair and snatched the receiver from her hand. "Hi, Larry. So happy you called."

"Would you like to go on a date with me tomorrow night? I was thinking maybe dinner and a Broadway show? There's a nice little French restaurant right next to my office building. I get off work at 5:30 so how about we meet there?"

Be still my beating heart! I would have been content with a sandwich at the Automat and a movie. This was the kind of date grown-ups went on. Trying to remain nonchalant, I replied, "That sounds OK," while frantically motioning to my mother to bring me a pad and pencil. "What's the address?"

Le Vert Gallant turned out to be a charming little bistro. I ordered onion soup, lobster tail, and chocolate mousse. Everything was delicious. I had to keep from wolfing it down so as not to come off as a crass glutton. Larry took my hand in his as we made our way to the theater, which made me deliriously happy. The show was *Jimmy Shine*, starring Dustin Hoffman in his Broadway debut. I struggled to focus on what was happening onstage because I was too busy thinking about what the post-performance action would be like.

I didn't have to wait long to find out. As we approached the corner of Seventh Avenue and West Forty-Eighth Street, the traffic light was about to turn red. While waiting for it to change to green, Larry leaned over and kissed me. I was over the moon six months before Neil Armstrong ever set foot on it.

Chapter 13

The Imposter Syndrome

Song: "The Great Pretender" sung by The Platters

In **February 2022, two of** the most popular shows streaming on Netflix were about imposters—*The Tinder Swindler* and *Inventing Anna*. *Swindler* is a documentary about an Israeli citizen named Shimon Hayut who used dating apps such as Tinder to dupe women into thinking he was the son of Lev Leviev, a fabulously wealthy diamond mogul. Passing himself off as Simon Leviev, he used a combination of charisma and greed to con several women out of a collective sum said to be $10 million.

Shonda Rhimes, famed for such TV megahits as *Grey's Anatomy* and *Scandal* is the creative force behind *Anna*. The nine episodes are loosely based on the real-life Anna Delvey, a Russian-born New Yorker who reinvents herself as a German heiress to her father's fortune. An uncannily gifted poseur, she peddles her dream of buying an expensive piece of prime Manhattan real estate to house what she has dubbed the Anna Delvey Foundation, only to wind up in prison on Rikers Island.

Their respective stories were so compelling that once I started watching, I could not stop. Though appalled by the deceitful, unprincipled methods these two talented grifters employ to obtain what they want, I was simultaneously fascinated by the unapologetic brazen behavior, self-confidence, and sheer chutzpah they displayed in pulling off their cons.

My binge-watching spree increased my appetite for more examples, so I turned to my computer. Not sure which combination of key words would yield the most productive searches, I figured some sort of personality trait probably accounted for most of their deviant doings and so began by typing "The Imposter Syndrome" in the Google search bar. A fair number of links came up; not one of them contained the answer I was seeking. Instead, they all defined the term in pretty much the same way: fear of being found out that you're not as accomplished as people think you are.

Something about this phrase resonated with me. I plunged further down the Google rabbit hole to try to identify the reason. Voilà! A posting from Canada's University of Waterloo maintained, "this phenomenon is based on intense, secret feelings of fraudulence in the face of success and achievement." That struck a chord. "You believe you have somehow cheated your way onto the podium...and don't deserve your success, even when you've worked hard for it." "Curious and curiouser," as Alice would say.

The clincher was this reference from Health.com. In their 1978 seminal paper, "The Imposter Phenomenon in High Achieving Women: Dynamics and Treatment Intervention," psychologists Pauline Rose Clance and Suzanne Ament Imes hypothesized there is a subset of high-achieving females who see themselves as intellectual frauds. They believe their successes are due to chance or lucky breaks despite being seen as very successful according to objective standards. Rose, who admitted to having experienced the phenomenon in graduate school, posited, "They are also pretty certain that unless they are prepared to go to gargantuan efforts to do so, success cannot be repeated. They are afraid that next time 'I will blow it.'"

Bingo! It finally dawned on me that I have experienced these symptoms more than once in my life, dating back to when I was about ten years old. By then, I had been taking piano lessons for three years and had become reasonably proficient. My mother felt I should sign up for Greenwood Inn's weekly guest talent show. Being somewhat of a ham, I obliged. I chose to perform "Dance of the Reed Flutes" from Tchaikovsky's *Nutcracker Suite*, a quick tempo piece with lots of flourishes. I heaved a sigh of relief when I made it to the end without any major faux pas.

Later that evening though, an unsettling sensation started building in the pit of my stomach when my mother began talking about playing another selection in the following week's show. I started wondering if I was just a one-hit wonder who wouldn't be able to reprise my performance next time out.

Two years later, I was chosen to give a short speech at our sixth-grade elementary school graduation. I never told my mother about it but didn't count on her ever finding out. I guess I underestimated the power of the neighborhood coffee klatch. Her good friend Joy Bernstein was a substitute teacher at PS 153. She called to congratulate my mom and asked if she wanted a ride to the ceremony.

At the time, I thought my reluctance to have her attend was because I was afraid that she'd feel embarrassed by having her child outshine her modest life accomplishments. Seeing that incident through the lens of Rose and Imes, gave me clearer insight.

A similar situation took place in high school. I was ranked

fourth in my graduating class of 1,216 students, making me the female student with the highest academic standing. Tradition called for the "highest boy and highest girl" to speak at commencement. To downplay this achievement, I decided that I would write a humorous talk because I knew I would feel more at ease behind the podium as the class clown rather than scholar. There was one catch: all commencement addresses had to pass the inspection of Ms. Tannenbaum, the AP English teacher. Thankfully, she loved it and gave me her blessing.

But it wasn't until midspring of 1969 that a full-blown episode of imposter syndrome hit me head-on. The semester started off on a high note. I was giddy from the whirlwind romance that had blossomed between Larry and me during intersession. Except for the Monday after our first date, we saw each other every other night while I was home. And the only reason for that outlier was I had promised my sister's friend Barbara I would go on a blind date with her cousin when we had both finished our finals.

On Tuesday, Larry got tickets for a Knicks home game at Madison Square Garden. It was the first time I had ever seen professional basketball, so it was pretty exciting—at least through halftime. I stood up and heartily cheered alongside Larry, hugging him with genuine enthusiasm whenever the Knicks scored. By the middle of the third quarter, my cheers were a little less "rah-rah" and my hugs were a bit more perfunctory. When it was clear the Knicks were so behind they couldn't possibly make a comeback, I made the mistake of turning to Larry and saying, "Probably makes sense for us to leave now so we can beat the crowd exiting the Garden."

The crestfallen look on his face indicated this was not a suggestion he had expected to hear. Nevertheless, he agreed. When we got back to my house, my mother was still up.

"Hope you two had a good time. I waited up to make sure you got home safely. Now that you're here, I'm going upstairs to bed." As soon as she was out of sight, Larry and I hightailed it to the couch and started making out. About five minutes into our session, a loud, unexpected sound came from above causing Larry to bolt upright, the proverbial deer in the headlights look on his face. "That's just my mom having one of her 'starts,'" I reassured him.

For as long as I can remember, my mother had been prone to occasional Tourette's Syndrome-like outbursts while she was asleep. They never roused her to a wakeful state, but they were loud and scary enough to startle those within hearing distance, hence the name my sister and I gave them. This was the first time it happened while I was entertaining a gentleman caller and it clearly rattled him. "Nothing's wrong," I hastened to reassure him. "Don't worry about her coming downstairs. She sleeps through them." When this failed to make him reassume his previously prone position, I switched tactics. "Someone seeing your expression right now would probably think you don't like me," I coyly teased. After a brief moment of silence, he blurted out, "Like you? Joan, I love you."

The rest of our week together was a whirlwind of long phone calls, movie dates, and heavy petting but we didn't go all the way until a month later when he flew up to Buffalo the weekend after my birthday. Since his flight wasn't due in until late evening, the plan was for him to stay with me in the dorm Friday night, then drive to Niagara Falls on Saturday for a day of sightseeing followed by dinner at John's Flaming Hearth, an upscale steak house whose signature dessert I recall being pumpkin pie ice cream. (Think Morton's The Steakhouse crossed with the Cheesecake Factory.) We would then spend a romantic night of lovemaking in a motel, and he'd drive me back to campus the next day before continuing to the airport for his flight back to New York City.

But as soon as I unlocked the key to my room that Bonnie and our third roommate, a sophomore named Anita, had graciously vacated for the evening, I discovered that absence does indeed make the heart—as well as genitalia—grow fonder. Granted, dorm rooms were never meant to be romantic boudoirs even when shared by two roommates. But this was the middle of the 1968-69 academic year—a banner one for college-bound baby boomers—and UB had experienced a rise in enrollment creating increased competition for on-campus housing.

Rooms meant for two had to be reengineered to accompany three by replacing one of the twin beds with a bunk bed and adding a third desk and dresser. Since I'd never slept in a bunk bed, I thought it might be fun to try it. Lucky for me, I won the coin toss and chose the cozier (and safer) bottom bunk because I wound up losing my virginity that night.

Our next rendezvous a month later more than made up for the surroundings on the night of my deflowering. I had signed up for the UB-sponsored spring break trip to the Bahamas. The university had booked a charter flight to Nassau and taken a block of double rooms at the Montague Beach Hotel, a once fashionable resort that was now a bit on the shabby side. When I told Larry about it, he decided to fly down and booked a room for the same time period. So, my luggage wound up vacationing in one wing while I took up residence in another.

That magical week in Nassau remains my favorite vacation of all time. Larry rented a little red sports car so we could tool around the island during the day. Early on in the week, we pulled off the road to take advantage of a scenic overlook. There we met a native

Bahamian named Prince who took a liking to us and volunteered to be our unofficial tour guide for the rest of our stay.

At night we gambled in the casino on Paradise Island and dined in upscale restaurants such as the Café Martinique, which was featured in one of the early James Bond movies. The fellow seated next to us one evening turned out to be Huntington Hartford II, heir to the A & P fortune and once ranked among the world's richest people. He owned the Ocean Club resort on Paradise Island, considered one of the fanciest hotels at the time and commissioned an Edward Durell Stone-designed modern art museum in NYC. We must have spent two hours with HH II while he regaled us with entertaining stories about his various exploits but sorry to say, he didn't offer to pick up our check.

As heady as that spring break vacation was, the best part about it was not having to con my parents with some elaborate cover story in order to keep them from finding out about their younger daughter's premarital tryst with an older man she had known for less than three months. Thank God for that because lacking the con artist mentality of scoundrels like Shimon and Anna, I would never have been able to pull it off!

On a more somber note, by the time I turned twenty in 1969, the antiwar movement had changed its tactics, with civil disobedience giving way to violent unrest. Building takeovers and unruly student protests were taking place at campuses all over the country. At UB, the turning point happened on March 19—the day before Larry's twenty-fourth birthday.

An estimated five hundred protesters occupied Hayes Hall, the administration building that housed the president's office, to give then president, Dr. Martin Mayerson, a list of demands: abolition of University accreditation for ROTC; an end to all defense research contracting; solidarity with the campus Black Student Union; support for the Buffalo Nine (who had been arrested on draft burning charges); and a pledge that construction would not begin on the proposed new Amherst campus without a fully integrated work force in place.

The raucous nature of the occupation was amplified when two students climbed the ivy-covered walls to the bell tower, where they proceeded to ring the clock bells continuously. After President Meyerson's negotiation efforts failed, he sought a court order to end the occupation. The protesters backed down when 150 Buffalo police officers arrived to enforce it.

Honestly, I wasn't surprised when the occupation occurred. After all, UB hadn't earned the reputation as the "Berkeley of the East" for nothing. As far back as May 1966, students had staged sit-ins and picketed Hayes Hall to protest the university's participation in administering a Selective Service Qualification Test to determine draft eligibility. The following year, Students for a Democratic Society (SDS) vowed to disrupt Dow Chemical Company from recruiting on campus and antiwar luminaries such as Allen Ginsberg and Jerry Rubin were frequent guest speakers. During the years that I was at UB, my friends and I had all become accustomed to the sight of the Buffalo K-9 corps patrolling the campus and the acrid smell of tear gas in the air.

What did surprise me was getting a call from WBFO's Henry Tenenbaum on the last day of winter, asking if I could rush over and cover the occupation of Hayes Hall. Up until that moment, I had only been a news reader; I had never kept a diary, written for my high school newspaper, or taken a course in journalism. Sure, I was able to sit down at my word processor and, relying on only an outline of my research notes, turn out submission-ready term papers, a skill that never ceased to amaze my roommates. Taking notes on the fly and turning them into a concise article while racing to meet a tight deadline? Hell, just thinking about it made me queasy. And when I had arrived on campus as a dewy-eyed freshman, I had visions of taking tea with the dean, not taking over his office. Would I be up to the task the station manager was asking of me?

But this was breaking news, and I didn't want to let him down. Grabbing my notebook and pen, I dashed across campus at breakneck speed. As I pushed my way through the ever-expanding crowd of angry, mostly male students, the last line from an Alfred Lord Tennyson poem flashed across my brain. "In spring, a young man's fancy lightly turns to thoughts of love." Well, spring was literally just around the corner and whatever was probably going through the minds of the young men facing conscription into a war they believed was immoral, probably had nothing to do with love. That's when I realized I had the lead-in for the piece.

Chapter 14

Wedding Belle Blues

Song: "Single Ladies (Put a Ring on It)" sung by Beyonce

"**Take a seat, Joan.** I want to talk to you about your coverage of the Hayes Hall riot."

I was in the WBFO station manager's office. It was a few days after the campus uprising had been quelled. Henry had called and asked me to meet with him. "I was intrigued by your reference to the Tennyson quote. Are you an English major?" Uh-oh, I immediately thought. He didn't like my literary approach to a hard news story.

"No, Psych. But my AP English teacher in high school was a big fan of his, so we read a lot of his work."

"Well, I doubt if any of my other reporters would have led off that way. Which is why I called you in." *Here it comes. I am about to get the ax.* "I think you're wasting your time here at WBFO just coming in and reading the news." Ouch! I slunk down in my chair. "I would like you to become our field reporter, effective with the start of the fall semester. Whadda you say?"

I said nothing and slunk down even farther. I was completely taken aback by Henry's offer. While I was relieved that I was not being fired, the thought of getting a promotion stirred up a different emotion: apprehension. Having no journalism experience, I was fearful I would not live up to Henry's confidence in me. Yet I realized that it might be a life-changing opportunity, one that could allow me to explore a career field I had never even considered. "Thanks, Henry. I am really flattered by your offer. Can I take some time to think about it and get back to you?"

"Sure. But I will need your answer before the term ends."

"Of course, no problem."

But there was a problem. All the thoughts and anxieties that bubbled up in response to Henry's offer were symptoms of the phenomenon that had been identified two decades earlier by Chance and Ames (which subsequently became known as Imposter Syndrome). Had I been aware of such an entity back then, perhaps I wouldn't have felt so bewildered and alone as I left Baird Hall and made my way back to my dorm.

The next few weeks passed by in a haze as I wrestled with my decision. The more I deliberated, the more I convinced myself I would not live up to Henry's expectations despite all evidence to the contrary. Then, of course, I had to factor Larry into the equation. By the end of our idyllic Bahamian getaway, it was clear our relationship was becoming serious. In fact, he had requested and been granted a transfer to a NYC reserve unit within weeks of meeting me, eliminating his need to make monthly visits to Batavia. Come senior year, most of my free time would likely be spent flying back home to visit him.

I managed to convince myself I could not in good conscience do justice to a demanding position as a radio reporter, a job for which I believed I was overwhelmingly underqualified, while juggling my academic and romantic lives. That was the angle I used in delivering my decision three weeks later—in writing rather than in person. Only I embellished it just a bit to make it seem more solid.

"Dear Henry, As much as I would like to accept your offer, I'm afraid I have to turn it down. I just got engaged (if only!) and my fiancé works in NYC. After talking it over, we've decided it would be best for me to transfer to Brooklyn College for my senior year. Yours truly, Joan Rubenfeld."

Of course, I did no such thing. But I began thinking that if I were to acquire formal education in communications, perhaps I could find a career niche in that field after all. As luck would have it, just before final exams I ran into another WBFO staff member, and we got to talking about our summer plans. He just happened to have a pamphlet in his backpack about a course being offered in Radio, Film, and TV at NYU and graciously handed it over to me.

One month later, I was at Loeb Student Center in Greenwich Village for the course orientation along with a diverse group of some twenty other students, including a nun and a priest. (No rabbi though. Which is too bad as I would have loved to slip in one of those "clergy bar mate" jokes here for a bit of David Sedaris-like humor.) It was an experiential curriculum designed to provide hands-on training. Each of us was tasked with writing, producing, casting, and directing a program in each medium; on any given day, you might be the cinematographer for a movie, the sound engineer for a radio broadcast, or on-air talent for a TV show.

The last possibility appealed to me the most because I'd been an inveterate TV fan for as long as I can remember. I fell in love with Howdy Doody from the moment I laid eyes on him. Of course, I didn't realize he was only an eighteen-inch marionette who talked and walked courtesy of Buffalo Bob, the cowboy clad-actor who manipulated his strings. Buffalo Bob's posse consisted of a motley crew of characters: Flub-a-Dub, Princess Summerfall Winterspring, and of course, that lovable lug, Clarabell, who communicated with the blast of an air horn that sent the kids in the peanut gallery into gales of laughter for no reason I could decipher. (To my ears, it sounded ominous, kind of like the shrill blast of sirens emitted by European police cars and ambulances.)

Though I never got to be one of the "peanuts," I did appear on another children's show, courtesy of a friend of my mom. She had an in with one of the producers of the *The Merry Mailman*, starring Ray Heatherton. If his name sounds familiar it's because his daughter, Joey, was a sexy singer/dancer/actress in the swinging 1960s. Unfortunately, she developed an eating disorder and substance addiction so was never able to develop the long-standing popularity of theatrical contemporaries such as Ann-Margaret, to whom she had often been compared.

Those were the days of live TV when commercials were often performed right on the set between different segments of the show. I seem to recall that on the day of my TV appearance, the show ran a toothpaste commercial. Even to this day, its catchy jingle remains imprinted on my brain:

Brusha, brusha, brusha, get the new Ipana
Brusha, brusha, brusha, it's better for your tee-eeth.

To fulfill the television production requirement, I created a takeoff of a popular cooking show called *The Galloping Gourmet*, hosted by a tall, slender debonair British chef named Graham Kerr. I decided my chef should be everything Graham was not and speak French with a terrible accent. I cast Tilak, a very dark-skinned, heavyset foreign student from Sri Lanka (the country formerly known as Ceylon) to play the role of Jean-Pierre and gave him a female assistant named Chantal played by Emily, a pretty Cornell co-ed who had cast me to play the lead in her production of *Medea*.

I wrote Jean-Pierre as a ladies' man who flirted with Chantal every chance he got, each time addressing her by the diminutive *mon petit chou* (my little cabbage), a uniquely French idiom for *sweetheart*. The episode I produced had him preparing a dish called "vegetables Provençale." It required Chantal to pick up a pair of very large, very ripe tomatoes and held them in front of her very ample, very perky breasts to demonstrate how juicy these ingredients needed to be while Jean-Pierre leered at her and smirked, *"Les tomatoes, ils sont tres grande, mon petit chou."* There was no way of missing the double entendre. As the pièce de résistance, I selected a treacly accordion track of "La Vie en Rose" as the show's final theme music and painstakingly timed it to run out at the precise moment the director gave the cue to fade to black. My attention to detail elicited great praise from the instructor as none of my classmates had thought to synchronize the music of their shows with the title sequences.

Tilak, Emily, and I spent a lot of time rehearsing and I began to suspect he had a crush on me. Unlike the character he played, Tilak was rather shy and unassuming so there were no smirks or leers in his arsenal of romantic ploys. But my suspicion was confirmed after the show was over when he gave me a trinket from his native country—a small ivory elephant on a slender gold chain. I was touched by his gesture but didn't want to lead him on. I put it around my neck and fingering it lovingly, told him, "Oh, it's absolutely beautiful. Thank you so much. I can't wait to show it to my boyfriend; he's coming tomorrow night to see me play the lead in Emily's show."

I was really excited about Larry coming to my debut as a

classical actress. But I could see from the way his eyes glazed over during the performance that he was not bowled over. He made it up to me by suggesting we go to a quaint, cozy Italian bistro a few blocks from Washington Square Park. Over veal parmigiana (his favorite dish) and veal saltimbocca (mine), we lamented it would soon be time for me to return to Buffalo. It had been nine months since we started to date and though neither of us had dated anyone else since, there had been no mention of a lifetime commitment either.

When I arrived back on campus to start senior year, all my close friends were either married or engaged. What's more, each of them had also committed to a definite career path following graduation: hospital administration (Ellen), audiology (Judy), and teaching (Jackie and Bonnie.)

As the semester progressed so did my fears about what I'd be doing and who I'd be doing it with come June. My anxiety went into high gear when I arrived home for Thanksgiving. Saturday night of that weekend, my parents were away visiting friends, so Larry and I took advantage of the empty house by retiring to my bedroom. When we heard the sound of the Chrysler pulling into the garage, we hastily prepared for their arrival. But the thought of returning to campus the next day without a ring on my finger made me jittery; so much so that when we were hastily putting our clothes back on, I couldn't resist issuing a veiled ultimatum along the lines of "Why buy the cow when you can get the milk for free?"

Wordlessly, Larry then headed downstairs while I remained behind to straighten up my room. I figured he planned to make a quick getaway to avoid having to face Ruth and Leon. Before the first of my second thoughts had even started to formulate in my mind, sounds of joy and cries of "Mazel tov" wafted upstairs. Wonder of wonder, miracle of miracles! He had gone down to ask my parents for my hand in marriage. While his approach may not have had the same dramatic flair as Jay-Z's mock proposal to Beyonce at the 2014 Met Gala, it nevertheless had the same effect on me. And elicited the same answer: "I do."

Photos

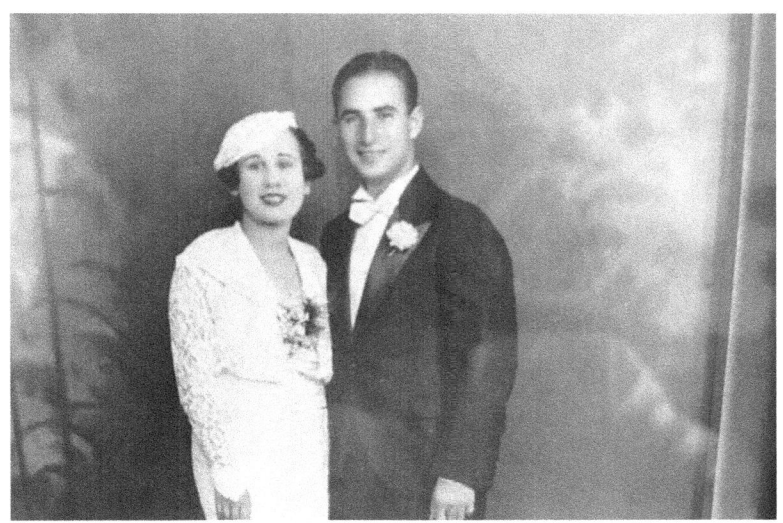

Wedding of Leo and Ruth Rubenfeld - August 31, 1935

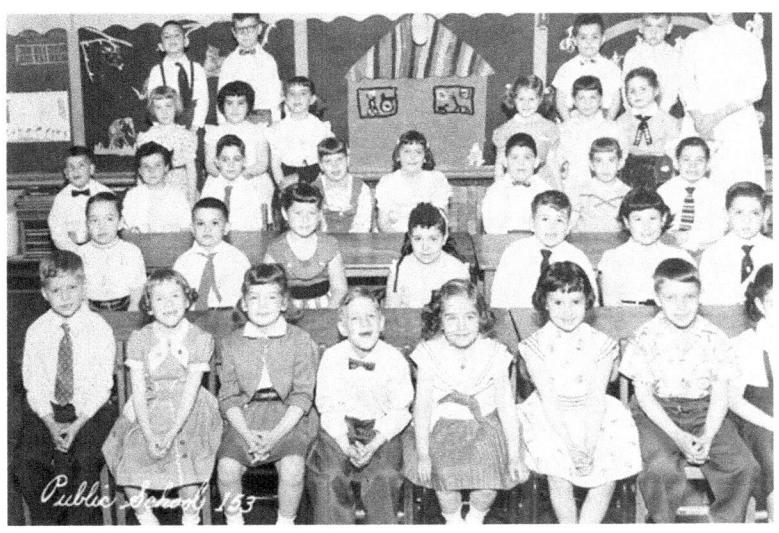

My start in academia (2nd row, 2nd from right)
- Kindergarten, PS 153

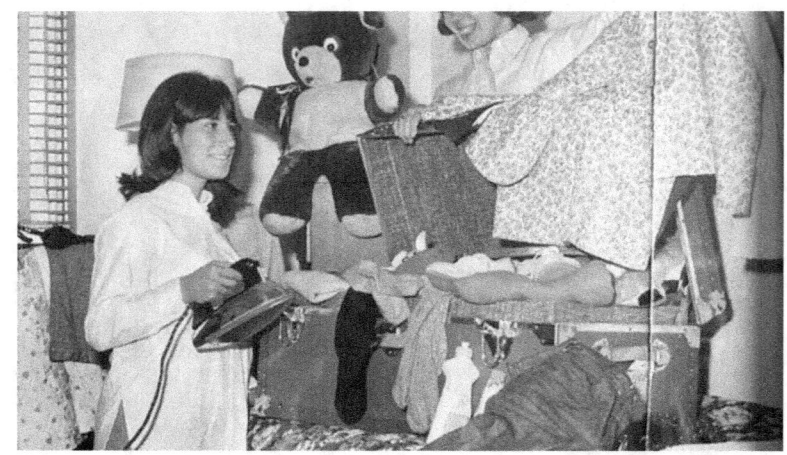

Moving In Day, September 1966 - Freshman Year at SUNY Buffalo
(Photo courtesy of Buffalo Evening News)

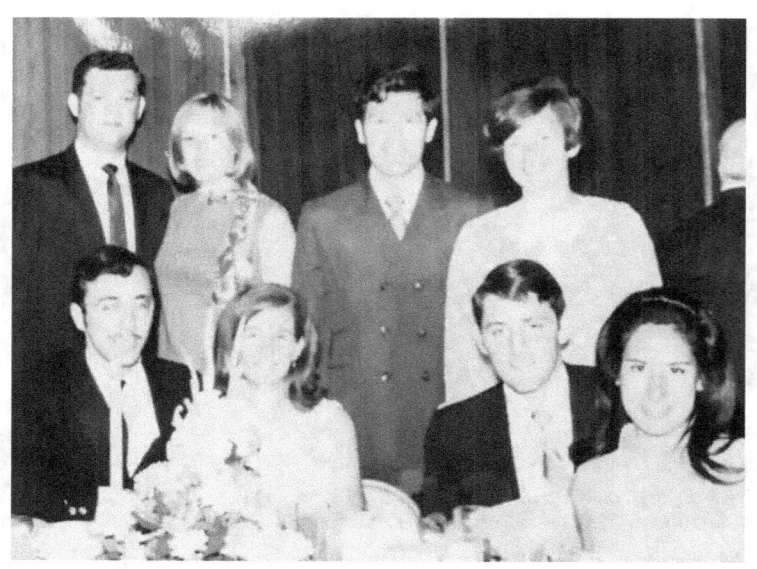

Four UB Gals at a June 1969 Wedding (clockwise starting with
me and Larry at bottom right: Jackie, Bonnie, and Judy.)
Ellen is missing as she was the bride!

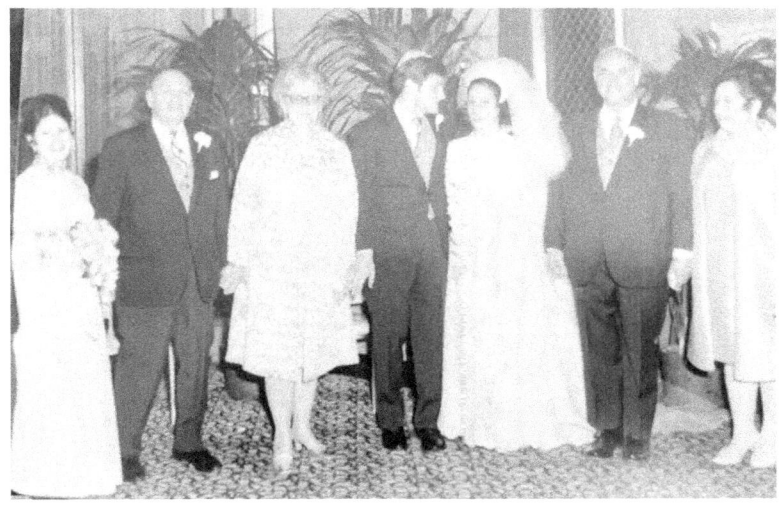

My wedding day, June 14, 1970
(left to right: My sister Susan, Larry's parents Henry and Paula,
Larry, me and my parents, Leo and Ruth)

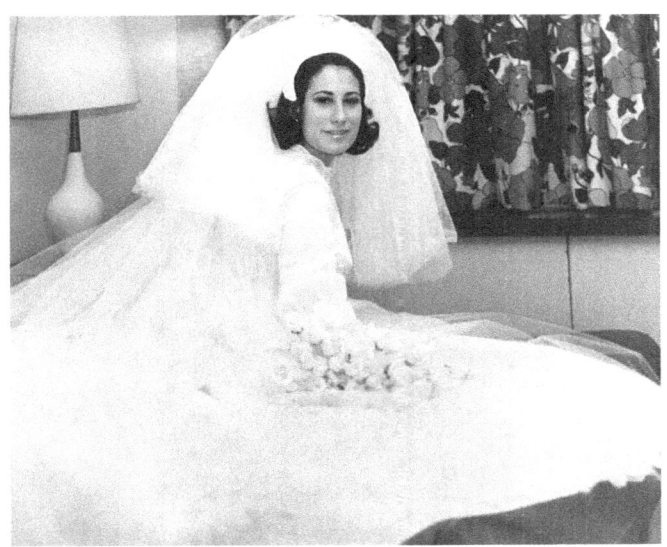

The Bride

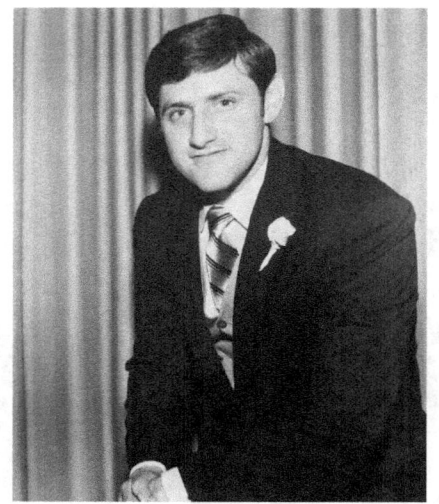

The Groom

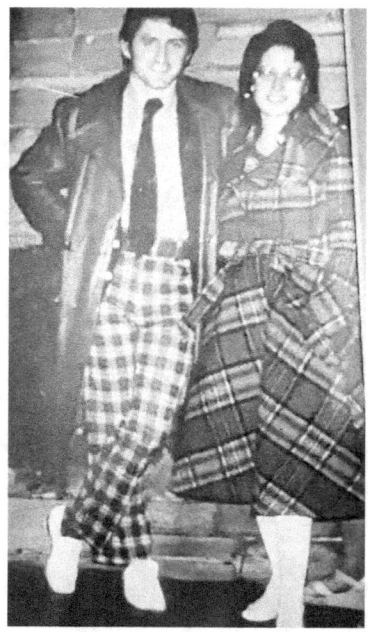

The "70s" called - they want their wardrobe back!

TO JOAN
WE STAYED TOGETHER THRU GOOD & BAD
SOME TIMES WERE HAPPY — OTHERS SAD

MY LIFE WITH YOU I CAN TRULY SAY
STILL GETS BETTER IN EVERY WAY

WHAT THE FUTURE HOLDS I DO NOT KNOW
I HOPE WELL BE TOGETHER THOUGH

MY LOVE MUST BE QUITE STRONG FOR YOU
BECAUSE MY OPTION I NOW RENEW.

A GIFT TO YOU AT A SPECIAL TIME
ACCOMPANIED BY MY HUMBLE RHYME

I HOPE IT WILL LAST
A SCENE FROM OUR PAST

ON THIS OUR EIGHTH ANNIVERSARY
A PICTURE OF THE NEW YORK LIBRARY.

LOVE,
Larry

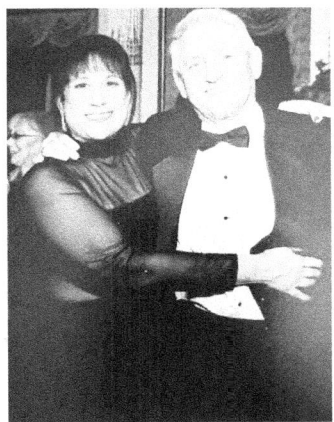

Celebrating my 8th anniversary with my very own poet laureate

Joan Liman, MD

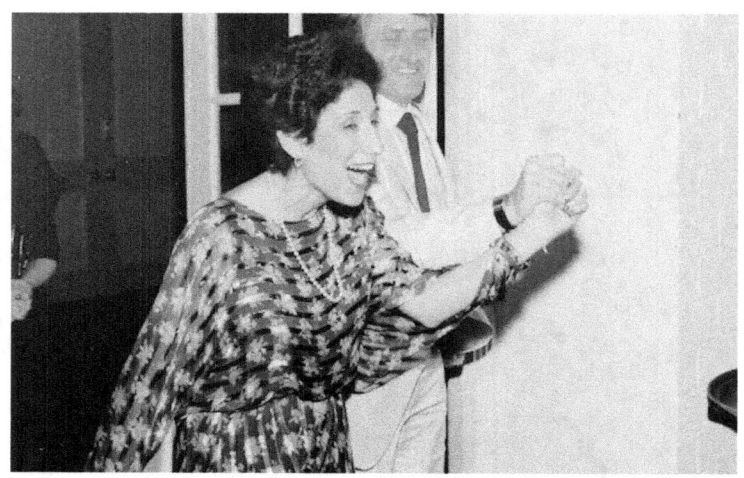

Surprise medical school graduation party - June 1983

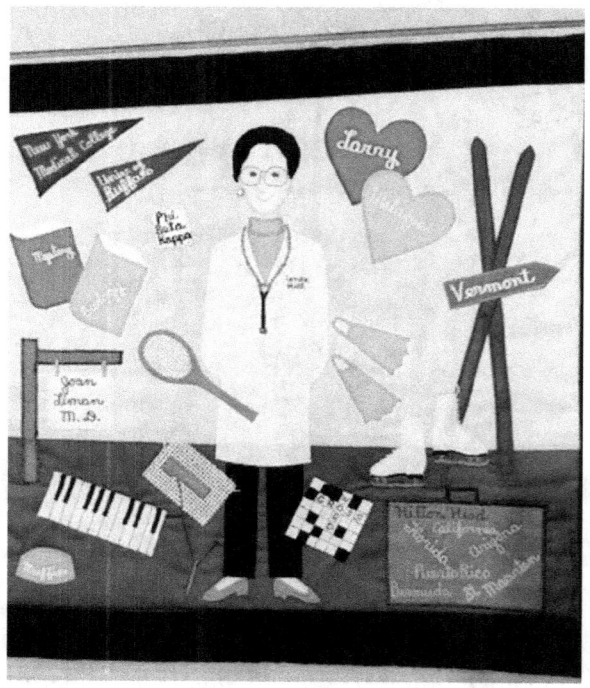

Favorite graduation gift - a hand-crafted collage

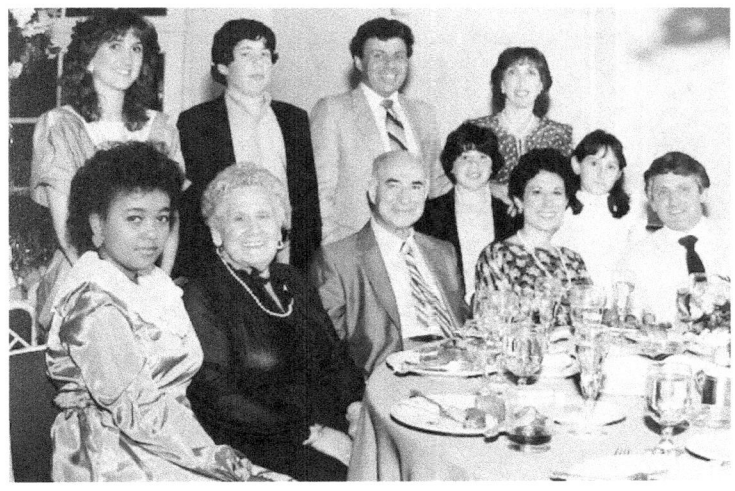

Family Portrait: Front row (sitting, right to left): My family and Melanie's beloved nanny, Charmaine
Middle row (standing): Melanie and Larry's nephew, Matthew
Back row: the rest of Larry's family (right to left: sister Bonnie, brother-in-law Sig, and their other two children, Jon and Jerilyn

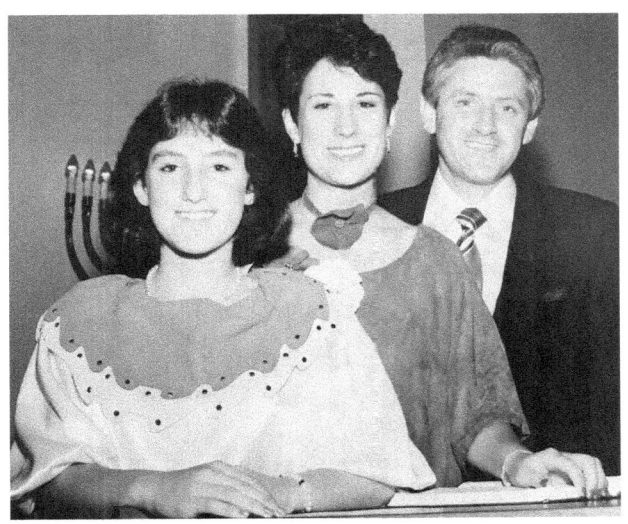

Melanie's Bat Mitzvah, October 1985

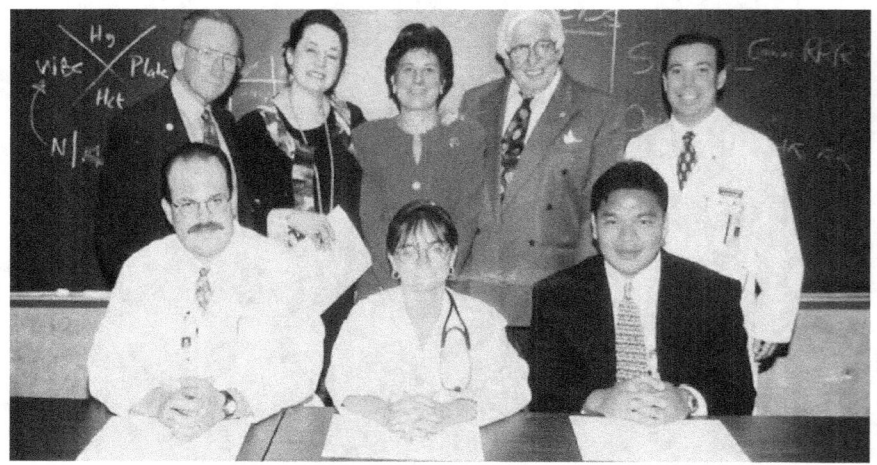

Arnold P. Gold, MD Foundation White Coat Ceremony at NJMS
(I'm flanked by him on my left and his wife, Dr. Sandra Gold,
on my right)

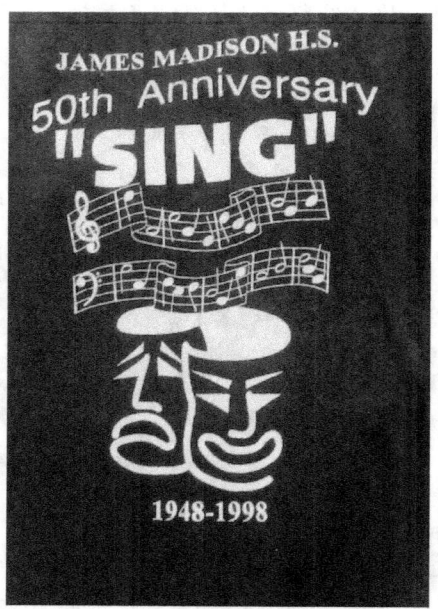

Commemorative T-shirt from 50th Anniversary of Madison "Sing"

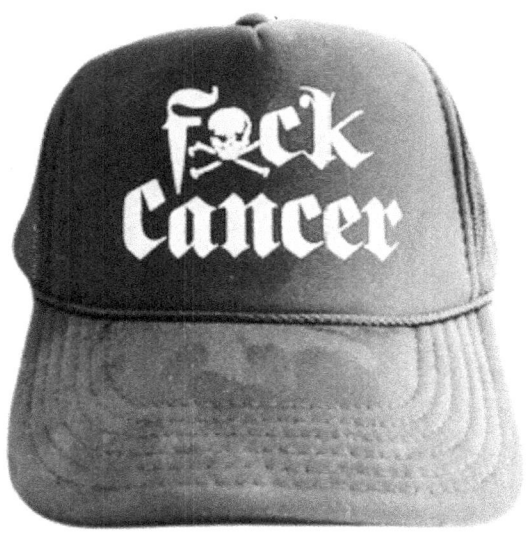

Self-explanatory!

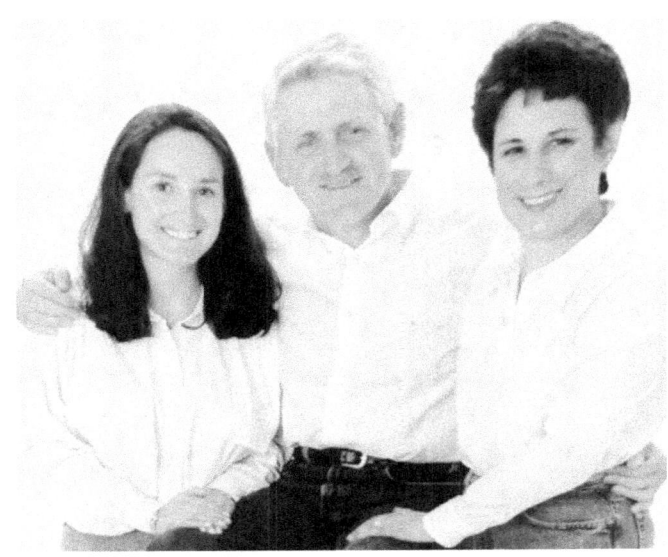

Post-breast cancer chemotherapy photo - First one without a wig

112

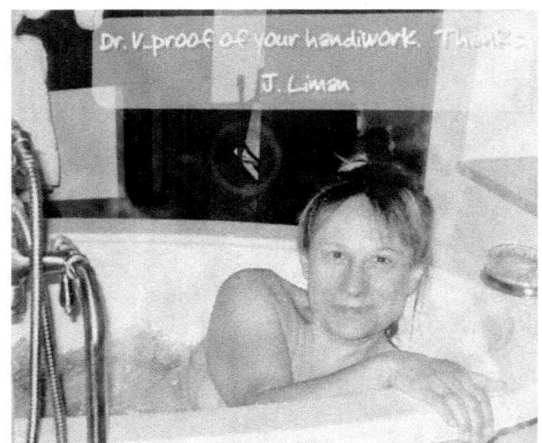

*Evidence of successful breast reconstruction by
my plastic surgeon, Dr. Vickery*

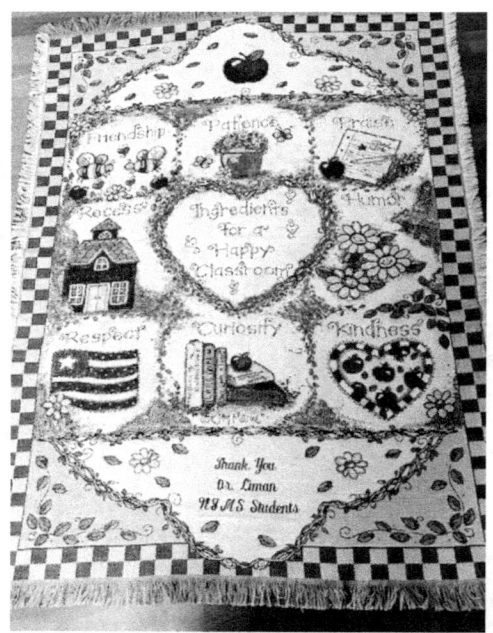

*Farewell gift from New Jersey Medical School student body
upon my departure, June 2001*

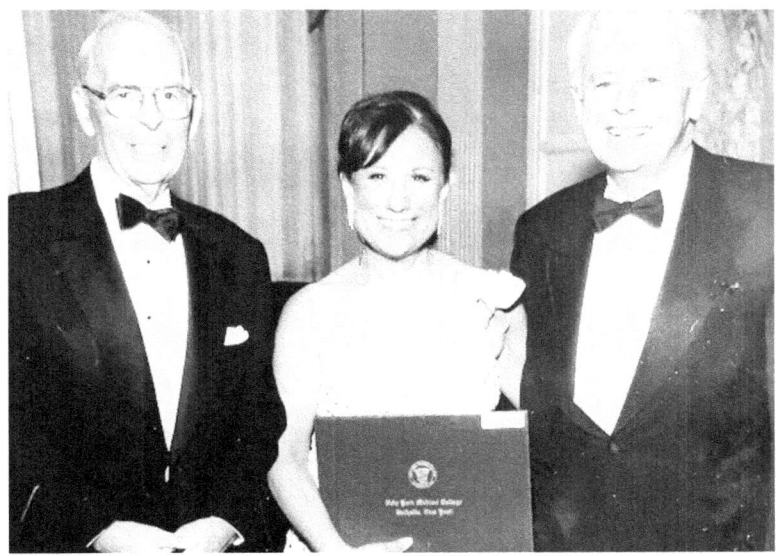

New York Medical College 30th Reunion. Left: Ralph O'Connell, MD,
Dean; Right: Karl Adler, MD., President

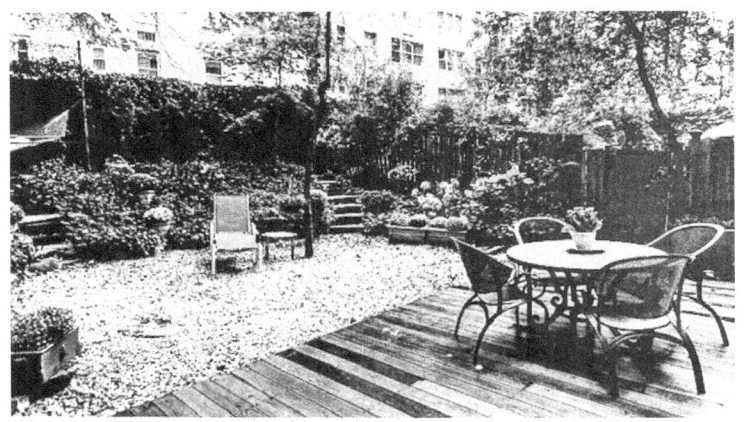

SPECTACULAR, MAGICAL, PRIVATE AND
EXCLUSIVE GARDEN OASIS

Garden, NYC pied-a-terre

Joan Liman, MD

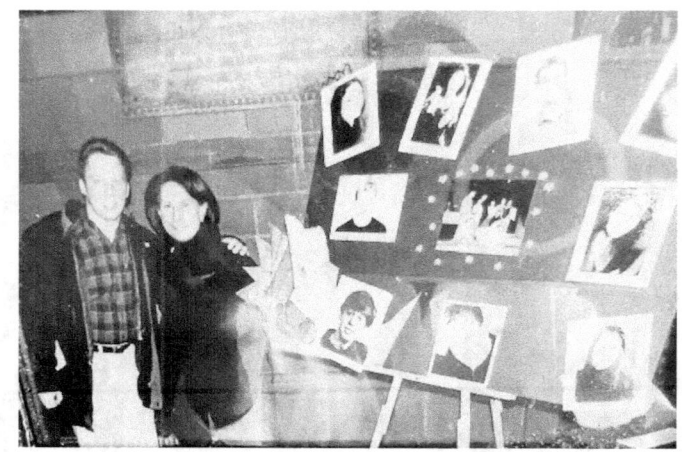

With my cousin Jeff Greenstein at my first musical production,
A Funny Thing Happened on the Way to the Manger

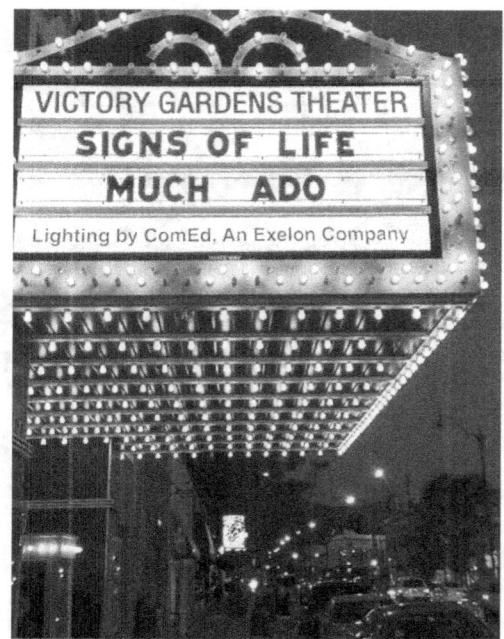

Chicago production of Signs of Life, *September 2013*

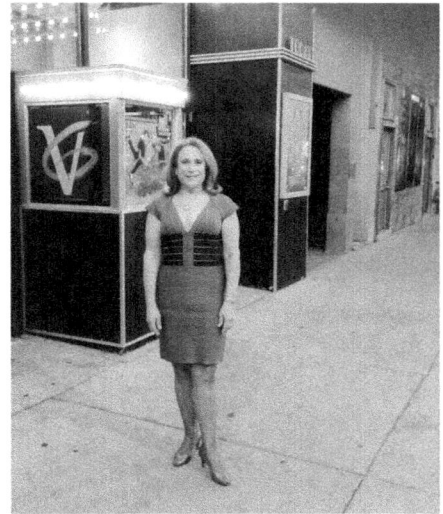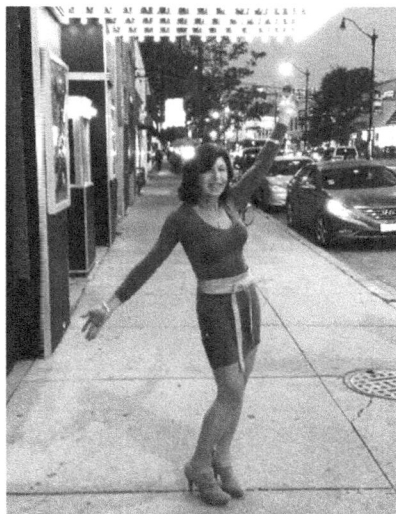

My friend Loni Figura (right) and me on opening night

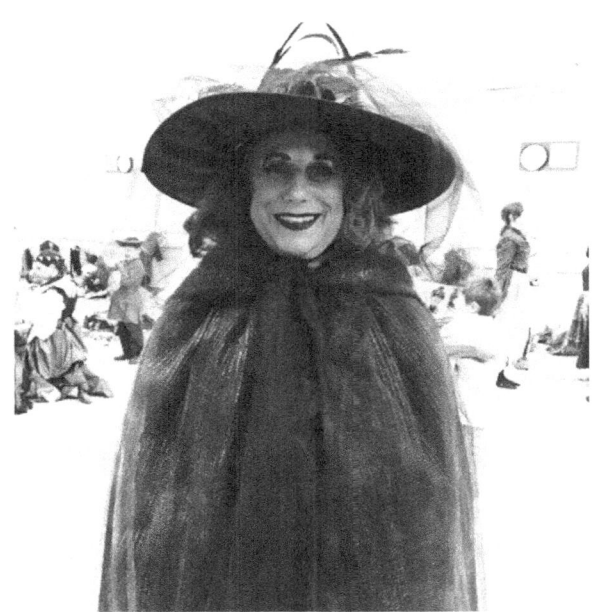

Me as the Wicked Witch of the West in
The Wizard of Oz *at Wayne, NJ "Y"*

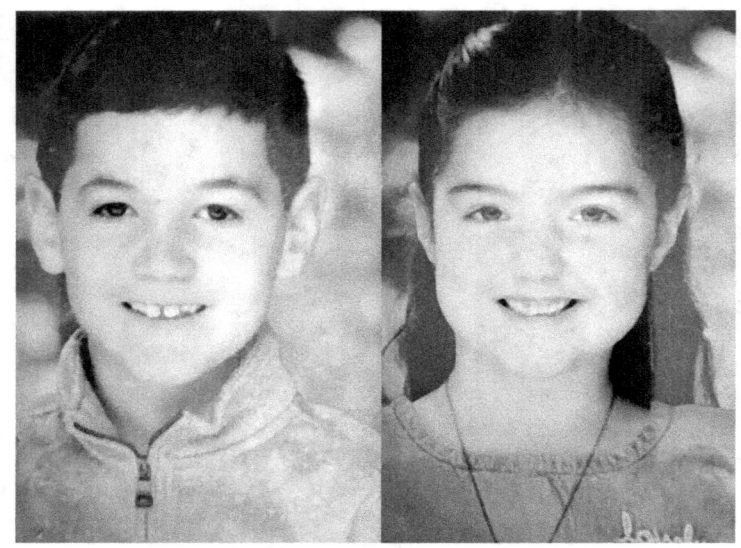

My grandchildren, Ryan and Marissa, in elementary school

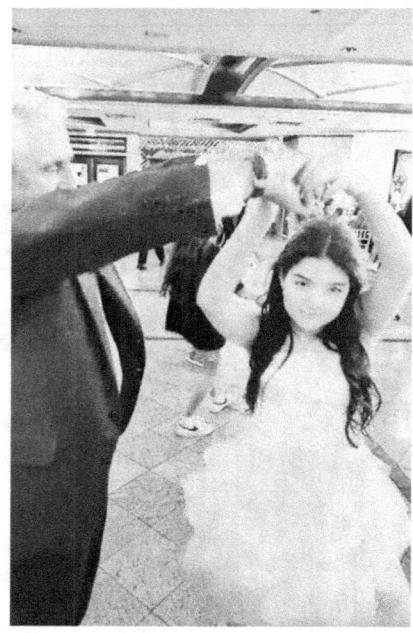

Marissa and "Pop Pop" at her bat mitzvah, November 18, 2023

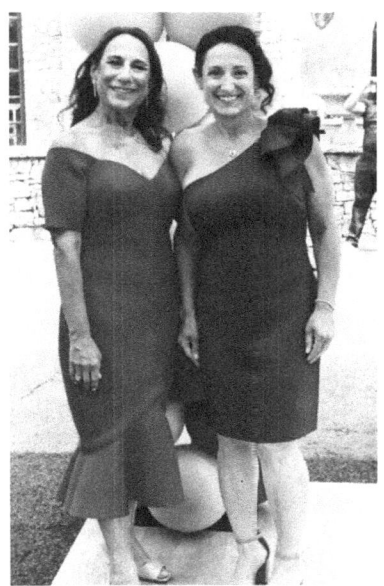

Me and Melanie at Ryan's bar mitzvah, May 20, 2021

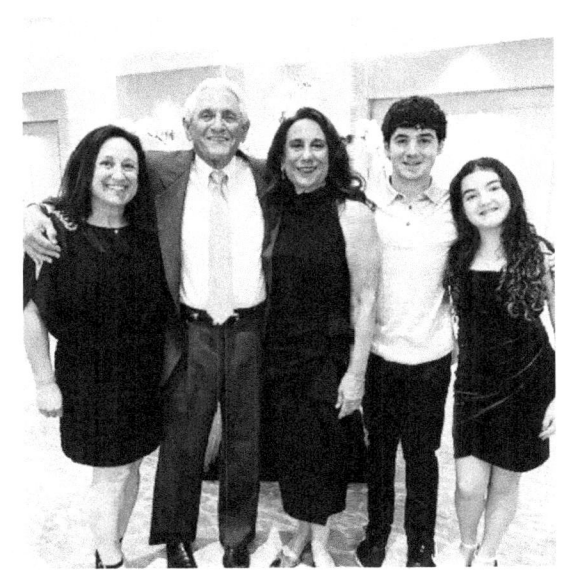

Celebrating my 75th birthday, February 17, 2024

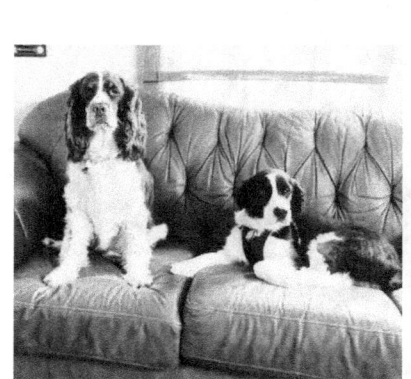
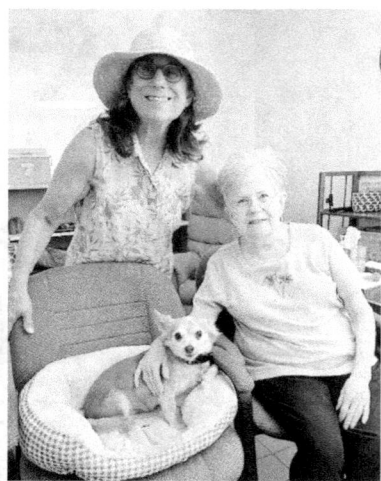

Canine cuties: my dog, Ariel, my 'grand dog' Reo,
and my sister's dog, Peanut.

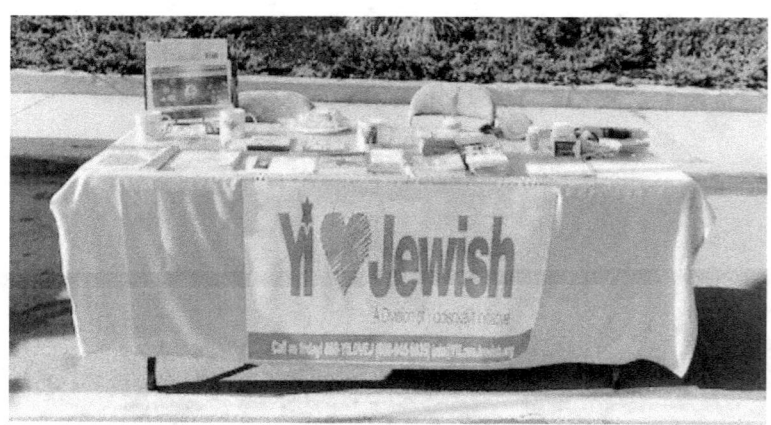

Yiddishkayt Initiative table, 2021, Annual Bagel Fest in Monticello, NY

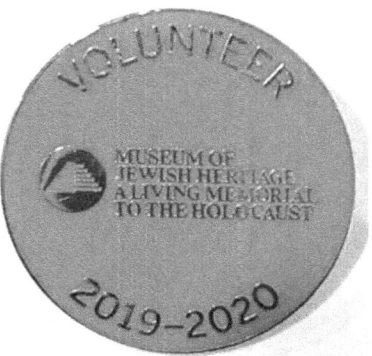

Gallery Educator Pin from NYC's Museum of Jewish Heritage docent program

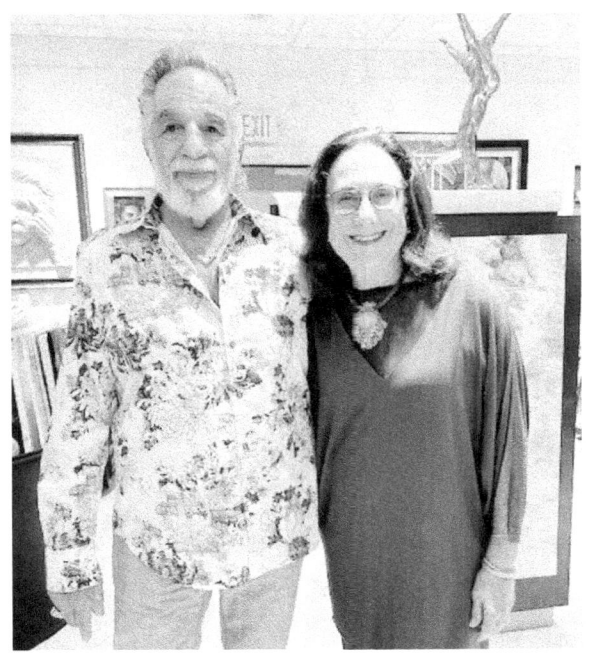

With world-famous Israeli artist Yaacov Heller at his gallery in Boca Raton, FL

Logo on one of my many anti-book banning T-shirts

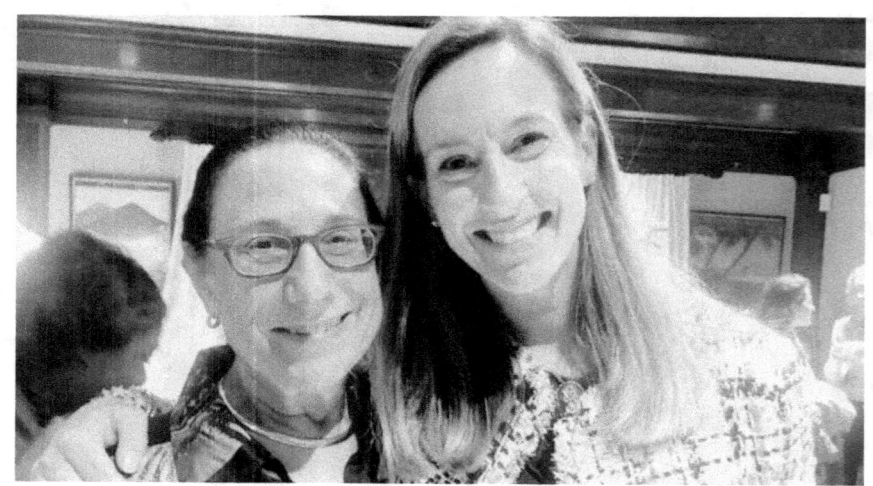

Fundraiser for NJ Congresswoman Mikie Sherrill

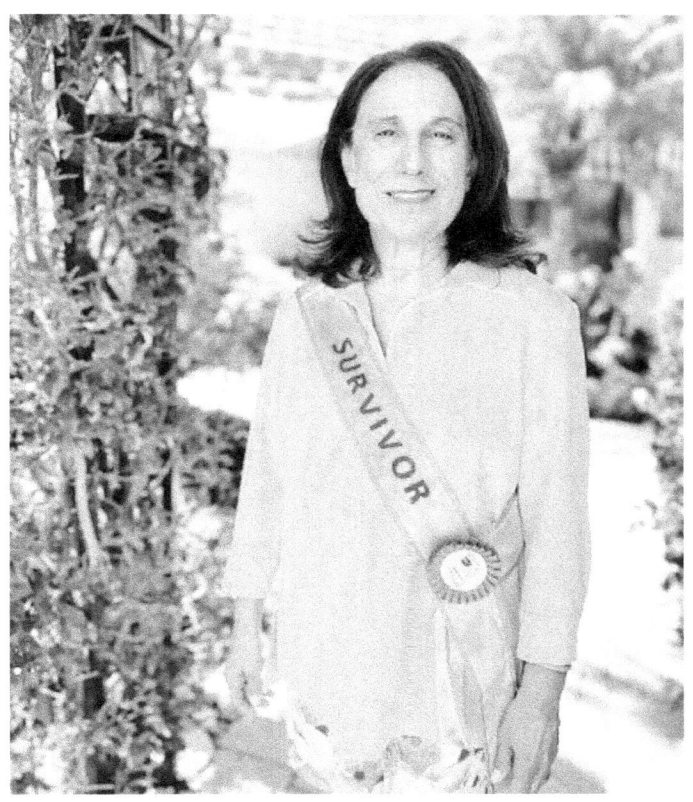

"I'm Still Standing" (Elton John) - Spring 2024

Chapter 15

Going to the Chapel

Song: "Going to the Chapel" sung by The Shirelles

Because we wanted to get married as soon as I graduated, wedding planning commenced almost immediately. The first person we consulted was Uncle Sam because Larry had to fulfill the US Army Reserve's annual summer camp training requirement. There was a small window of opportunity between UB's scheduled June 1970 commencement date and July 1, which was the earliest date that he could be called up.

June being the most popular month for weddings, most of the catering places within our price range had already been booked months in advance. Through the beauty parlor grapevine, my mother heard from someone, who heard from someone whose son had recently gotten married at what was then called The International Hotel at JFK Airport. She thought it would make a convenient locale for the 160 or so wedding guests on our list, almost all of whom lived in Brooklyn, Queens, or Long Island.

Normally, I would have opted for a more upscale setting. Nevertheless, since Larry and I probably would never have met each other had it not been for that fateful day at an airport, I was happy to go along with it. The only available weekend date was Sunday, June 14. This presented somewhat of a dilemma as Bonnie and her fiancé, Scott, had picked that date months ago. Taking it meant that all our mutual friends would most likely attend her wedding instead of mine.

With the end of the semester fast approaching, I didn't have time to fly home and scout out other sites. I told my parents to book it. Likewise, I didn't have the luxury of leisurely shopping for a custom-made wedding gown as I wouldn't be able to schedule repeated fittings. Customarily, the mother of the bride is the parent most involved in this process. In my case, the honor was reserved for my father given his many years of experience in bridal couture.

On the Saturday of spring break, before I had to return to campus, he took me to the showroom of the wedding gown manufacturer he represented. The company was closed on weekends, so we had the entire place to ourselves. He rifled through rack after rack of floor-length white dresses, selecting ones he thought would look good on me. I managed to find one that fit perfectly except for the length. My dad grabbed a pincushion from the nearest sewing machine table, got down on his knees, and pinned up the dress in one or two places so the seamstress could hem it when she came in on Monday.

He then steered me to a different part of the showroom and proceeded to rummage through a large container of bridal headpieces. Finally, he picked one out and with a satisfied smile, placed it on top of my head.

"This style is really in fashion now. All my buyers stock them." He turned me around so I could see myself in the mirror. Between the high-necked, empire-waisted, long-sleeved, lace-bedecked sat-in dress and the snug-fitting, pillbox-like chapeau with tapered side pieces that flanked my forehead, I looked as if I'd channeled Jackie Kennedy playing Julie Andrews as Queen Guinevere in *Camelot*.

My sister was to be my only bridal attendant, so Dad suggested I pick out a dress in any color I liked, and bring it home in a range of sizes for her to try on. A canary yellow floor-length number with orange, yellow, and green embroidery around the waistband called out to me. He put it in a garment bag along with the wedding gown and we headed home. Total time spent choosing and trying on attire for the bridal party: less than fifty minutes.

The rest of the to-do list was left to my mother as I had to return to Buffalo for the final weeks of my senior year. She commandeered my sister to assist her in ordering invitations, hiring a band, and drawing up the seating chart. When it came to the menu, I gave them one stipulation: the wedding cake had to be chocolate and instead of the traditional bride-and-groom cake topper, I wanted a toy model of an airplane sporting the "AA" logo.

While my entire family held down the fort in Brooklyn, I divided my time between my dorm room and the university library to prepare for the final set of exams of my undergraduate career. As the weather gradually warmed up, I contemplated a change of scenery and decided to move outside to the grassy area surrounding the fountain in front of Norton Hall. My plans for alfresco studying, however, were soon thwarted by a sudden change in climate and I am not talking about the meteorological kind.

Chapter 16

Ohio

Song: "Ohio" sung by Crosby, Stills, Nash, and Young

It was the first week of May. Like most of my student counterparts around the country, final exams loomed ahead of us. But studying for them became a moot point on May 4, 1970. On that day, Kent State University students protesting the bombing of Cambodia by United States military forces, clashed with Ohio National Guardsmen on the Ohio campus. In the ensuing melee, Guardsmen opened fire, killing four students and wounding nine others. That skirmish became the focal point of a nation already deeply divided by the Vietnam War.

The protest had started a few days earlier. On the evening of May 1, several incidents occurred, including rocks and bottles being thrown at police officers and the lighting of bonfires. These incidents led to the closure of bars by authorities before normal closing time to reduce alcohol consumption. Eventually students, other antiwar activists, and common criminals began to break windows and loot stores.

A state of emergency was declared on May 2, and National Guard members were called up to help maintain order. Upon their arrival, the soldiers found the Reserve Officer Training Corps (ROTC) building on fire even though university officials had already boarded up the structure and were planning to raze it. The soldiers resorted to tear gas to disperse the protesters.

By May 3, approximately one thousand National Guard soldiers were on the Kent State campus. Tensions remained high, and Ohio Governor Rhodes further escalated the situation by accusing the protesters of being unpatriotic. Some Kent State students assisted local businesses and the city in cleaning up damage from the previous night's activities, but other students and nonstudents continued to hold protests.

On May 4, a Monday, classes resumed while antiwar protesters scheduled a noon rally on the campus. University officials attempted to ban the gathering, but this proved unsuccessful. As the protest began, National Guard members fired tear gas at the demonstrators but due to wind, it proved ineffective. Some of the protesters threw the canisters, along with rocks, back at the soldiers; some yelled slogans, such as "Pigs off campus!" at them.

Eventually seventy-seven Guardsmen advanced on the protesters with armed rifles and bayonets. Protesters continued to throw things. Twenty-nine of the soldiers, purportedly fearing for their lives, eventually opened fire. The gunfire lasted just thirteen seconds, although some witnesses contended that it lasted more than one minute.

The Kent State shootings escalated protests across the country. Many colleges and universities canceled classes for the remainder of the academic year in fear of violent demonstrations erupting on their campuses. Ohio State University dismissed its spring quarter classes in early May and other Ohio schools followed suit. The various protests drew to an end as President Richard Nixon began to withdraw US soldiers from North and South Vietnam. With the signing of the Paris Peace Accords in 1973, which basically ended US involvement in the Vietnam War, the protests drew to a formal close, bookending a turbulent chapter of American history.

Since then, Kent State has held a commemoration ceremony every May 4 on the university campus. With the passage of time, the exact day and date of the tragedy faded from my memory; in mid-April of 2024, however, it came flooding back as I watched news reports of campus unrest growing exponentially across the United States. Iran launched a drone attack over Israel, escalating Israel Defense Forces' efforts to destroy Hamas in a war precipitated by the terrorist group's savage October 7, 2023 attack against the world's only Jewish state.

I couldn't shake the sense of déjà vu that only grew heavier as April turned into May. By then, college administrators found themselves in a face-off with students protesting a faraway war as they sought to preserve the latter's right to free speech while struggling to avoid campus shutdowns and canceling commencements for the class of 2024—the same class that in many cases had been cheated of donning caps and gowns at high school graduations because of the COVID-19 pandemic. I worried that protestors would hijack the day of the Kent State massacre to stage a nationwide event designed to demonstrate their unity and willingness to put themselves in harm's way in support of their goals. To my knowledge, May 4 came and went without any reports of loss of life on either side of the protest lines (although regrettably, serious injuries most likely occurred) and campus encampments started to be dismantled, some by local police and others voluntarily.

Nevertheless, the decidedly anti-Semitic trope that had characterized the protests continued to reverberate with increasingly more anecdotes from Jewish students being reported in various news outlets. The headline of a May 22 article in *The New York Times* captured the zeitgeist right before the start of Memorial Day weekend: On Campus, a New Social Litmus Test: Zionist or Not. It read in part:

"Some Jewish students on campus believe these dynamics amount to a kind of litmus test: If you support Palestine, you're in. If you support the existence of or aren't ready to denounce Israel, you're out. And they say this is not limited to pro-Palestinian protests. It is, instead, merely the most pointed form of a new social pressure that has started to drip down from the public square onto the fabric of everyday campus life, seeping onto spaces that would seem to have little to do with Middle East politics—sports clubs, dance competitions, sororities, and fraternities, even libraries."

Mention of the public square stirred up memories of disturbing photos I had seen some three months earlier while doing research for a 451 Avengers* talkback scheduled to follow the Boca Raton International Jewish Film Festival's screening of the Jeremy Irons-narrated Hitler documentary, *The Books He Didn't Burn*. Thoroughly disquieting, they recalled the events of May 10, 1933 when right-wing students at Germany's Wilhelm Humboldt University took books from its library, including works by Albert Einstein and Sigmund Freud, and threw them into a bonfire while giving the Nazi salute, coupled with a wide- angle shot of tens of thousands of people crowded into the plaza of the Berlin State Opera to hear Joseph Goebbels pronounce "the era of extreme Jewish intellectualism is now at an end."

But the most haunting takeaway from my research were the prescient words of the Jewish-born German philosopher, Heinrich

Heine (1797-1856):

> *"Wherever they burn books, they will also, in the end, burn human beings."*

South Florida grassroots organization founded to increase awareness of book banning and promote efforts to stop it.

Chapter 17

First Comes Love,
Then Comes Marriage...

Song: "Makin' Whoopee" sung by Eddie Cantor

The remainder of my senior year unwound in a surreal manner. Final exams were canceled. A somber mood pervaded the campus as students packed up their belongings and cleared out of the dorms, tightly hugging each other and bidding tearful good-byes. No announcement had been made as to whether the June commencement would be held as originally scheduled.

For many seniors, farewells proved to be the very last ones to classmates we'd lived, studied, commiserated, and partied with for the past four years. The culmination of our college careers would forever be associated with the grim photos being flashed on television cameras and adorning newspaper front pages for the next few weeks, making it difficult for me to take pleasure in what should have been one of the happiest times in my life—the countdown to my wedding day.

Though plans for the ceremony and reception had all been finalized, there were still a few last-minute details for me to attend to, namely finding a job and getting a marriage license—in that order. The tragic events in Kent, Ohio convinced me I'd made the right decision when I abandoned the idea of pursuing medicine as a career. The graphic images of unarmed students being roughed up and gunned down in a Midwestern college town made me realize I would have felt very uneasy setting foot on any university campus in the fall. Remembering how much I had enjoyed my NYU summer course and the easy A it earned me, I thought I'd try my hand at finding an entry level job in communications.

Sporting my Phi Beta Kappa key, I made the rounds of TV and radio stations in Manhattan, but I never even made it past the receptionists. Wanting to have a job offer by the time I got back from my honeymoon, I turned to the classified ads section in the Sunday *New York Times*. Back then, it was common practice to separate listings into male and female openings. Positions requiring high-level skill sets and offering more than minimum wage salaries were less likely to appear in the "Females Wanted" column. A listing for a "personnel interviewer" at the NYC headquarters of Metropolitan Life Insurance Company required a minimum of a bachelor's degree and "good communication skills."

If I couldn't land a job interviewing celebrities and heads of state, I convinced myself this would be a close second. I sent off a résumé and cover letter and was delighted to get a phone call a few days later from the head of Human Resources, inviting me in for a meeting. Shortly thereafter, I received a letter in the mail offering me the position. The salary was a paltry seventy-four hundred dollars a year but there was a decent benefit package, including one meal a day in the company cafeteria, which had the distinction at the time of being the country's largest nonmilitary feeding establishment. (Who says there's no such thing as a free lunch?) I checked off Find a Job on my countdown list and proceeded to tackle the next item.

In order to obtain a marriage license back then, it was standard practice throughout the country to require couples to undergo blood testing to detect genetic disorders and venereal disease, most commonly syphilis. The roots of such an invasive mandate date back to England in the 1880s. Francis Galton, half cousin to Charles Darwin, coined the term *eugenics* (good birth) to propose selectively breeding for positive traits "to produce a highly gifted race of men by judicious marriages during several consecutive generations" and eliminate undesirable traits such as physical or mental disabilities. Hitler proudly admitted to following the laws of several American states that allowed for the prevention of reproduction of the "unfit." (Black 2003.)

A famous legal case involving eugenics was the 1927 Supreme Court case of Buck v. Bell, in which the state of Virginia sought to sterilize a feeble-minded woman who had given birth to a baby out of wedlock (it was suggested she had been raped.) In ruling against Buck, Justice Oliver Wendell Holmes Jr. opined:

"It is better for all the world, if instead of waiting to execute degenerate offspring for crime, or to let them starve for imbecility, society can prevent those who are manifestly unfit from continuing their kind."

This was still the prevailing moral milieu in the late 1930s, prompting US Surgeon General Thomas Parran to institute a public health campaign based on the premise that *"premarital testing was necessary to inform the potential marriage partner of the risk of contracting a communicable disease, and to reduce the risk of birth defects associated with syphilis."*

That's a quick rundown of how I found myself standing in line on an unusually hot morning at 125 Worth Street in downtown Manhattan, the building that housed the NYC Department of

Health where premarital blood testing was performed. The exam was generally referred to as the Wassermann test, even though August von Wassermann was one of three scientists who developed the serological procedure for detecting syphilis. I was informed it would take a few days to mail me the results, but my wedding date was still a few weeks away, so I assumed the delay wouldn't pose any problem.

As June 14 drew closer, I began worrying because I still hadn't received anything in the mail. The reason why became clear when Dr. Feldbau, our courtly, European-born family physician, made an unexpected house call about ten days before the wedding.

"I'm afraid I have some upsetting news for you, my dear. Your blood test came back positive for syphilis."

"WTF," I mumbled under my breath. Regaining my composure, I stood up straight and looked him right in the eye. "That can't possibly be true. I've never had sex with anyone other than my fiancé and I'm pretty sure he has been faithful to me from the day we met." (After all, Larry had told me he loved me within six days after our first date.)

"It's possible the test result is wrong. The only way to know for sure is to go back down to Worth Street and get retested."

Unbeknownst to me, individuals with a history of hepatitis often tested positive on the Wasserman test because of cross reactions, so more refined screening needed to be done to rule out whether I did in fact have syphilis. Happily, I did not. The license was issued in the nick of time and on Flag Day, 1970, we were patriotically pronounced man and wife according to the powers vested by the state of NY in the rabbi who officiated at Larry's bar mitzvah.

Our first home as a married couple was a lower-level garden apartment in Ledgewood Terrace, a brand-new complex located in the blue-collar town of Little Ferry, New Jersey. Only twenty minutes or so by bus from Manhattan's Port Authority Terminal, it allowed for an easy commute to my office on East Twenty-Third Street and Madison Avenue. An interesting assortment of people could be found roaming the terminal's first floor that summer of 1970, from waiflike figures with shaved heads in saffron-colored robes, peacefully chanting "Hare Krishna, Hare Krishna," accompanied by the tinkling of handheld cymbals, to more robust individuals wearing camouflage-like outfits, sporting a variety of Afro-inspired hairdos, carrying armloads of newspapers and shouting, "*Panther News*, here. Check it out. Check it out. Come get your *Panther News*."

I was one of a dozen personnel interviewers. Each occupied an open-air, six-foot-by-six-foot cubicle, with room for only a desk and two chairs. The top half of the cubicle's walls were made of glass. Three assistant directors sat side by side along the back wall in slightly larger versions of our offices and the department director oversaw the entire operation from his spacious (maybe ninety square feet) corner suite. There was no privacy whatsoever. Talk about Big Brother watching. It was somewhat disconcerting at first, but gradually I got used to it.

Our division was responsible for hiring lower-level employees such as file clerks, typists, etc. While the job application was pretty pro forma, the intake sheet used to record our assessment of a candidate's suitability for employment contained one category that by today's standards would be verboten: What provisions have you made to provide for childcare while you are at work?

The overwhelming majority of our applicants were female, many of them single mothers from NYC's lower socioeconomic levels. Company protocol required that unless an individual already had a sound plan in place as well as a backup arrangement in case of emergencies, the application would automatically be rejected no matter how qualified (or in some cases, overqualified) the applicant. The same conundrum applied to people with disabilities. No matter how highly they scored on the mandatory aptitude test, these individuals were almost always precluded from consideration for employment.

Mind you, the year was 1970. The feminist movement was still in its infancy and the concept of offering workplace accommodations for people with disabilities had yet to be promulgated. I began to wonder whether there might be ways to address these employment inequities. What if MetLife were to establish an on-site day care center so parents could touch base with their children on their breaks or lunch hours? And speaking of lunch, the in-house food service could be expanded to offer hot breakfasts for their children, eliminating a mad morning rush to get them fed and still get to work on time, no doubt improving employee punctuality. Plus, there was an in-house employee health service that even included a dental office so medical attention would be readily available in case of an emergency.

Similarly, what if the configuration of the clerical floors were to be reengineered so that file cabinets were no longer started at floor level but were built so that a wheelchair could be rolled underneath them, eliminating the need to bend down throughout much of the workday? This would not only benefit wheelchair–bound employees but would help decrease the incidence and prevalence of back pain in able-bodied personnel, a very common reason for work absences. What about allowing the use of headphones by sensory-challenged people who found it difficult to stay on task if ambient noise levels were too distracting?

The concept of workplace day care centers eventually began to gain wider acceptance as studies showed how companies that offered this benefit had better attendance, greater productivity, and improved morale. However, even today they are still not as common in the US as they are in other parts of the world and it was not until 1990 that the Americans with Disabilities Act was passed, prohibiting discrimination based on disability.

Discouraged by what I saw as unnecessary restraints on my ability to hire the best person for the job, and feeling powerless to do away with them, one year into the job I knew I was not cut out for the corporate world. Around the same time, my father had a heart attack while on one of his business trips to Boston and Larry had to fly there to drive him back home. Dad's brush with mortality made both of us realize he might die before ever having grandchildren as my sister was still single with no marital prospects on her horizon. So, when Larry began talking about starting a family, I was all in. Right before my twenty-third birthday, I learned I was pregnant.

Since paid maternity leave was more like an oxymoron in 1972 than a widespread practice and I didn't plan to return to MetLife. I eventually gave notice I'd be leaving at the end of May. Ledgewood Terrace did not allow children, so we initiated house-hunting right away. We found a modest starter home on a quarter-acre plot in northern New Jersey, right around the corner from an elementary school. Moving day was set for a week in late June.

The morning of the move, we woke up to a full-blown hurricane bearing down. Thinking back, it might have been a harbinger of some of the turbulent times that lay ahead of us. But the move took place as scheduled. I spent the next three months happily picking out a layette, babyproofing the house and turning one of the three bedrooms into a nursery. Yet, I still felt something was missing from my life.

It was the only summer since I was sixteen that I had not been working or going to school and I didn't have any close friends or relatives nearby, so I was alone most of the time. Larry left the house around 7:00 a.m. and usually didn't walk in the door until twelve hours later, leaving me with no one to talk to in between, other than a quick hello to a neighbor or making small talk with the fatherly gentleman who worked the deli counter at our local Foodtown. My mother couldn't come out to visit during the week unless someone drove her, and my sister had never bothered learning how to drive since she was able to commute by subway to her high school teaching job.

I began to feel very isolated and questioned whether Larry and I had made the right decision by moving to suburbia where public transportation was woefully inadequate and sidewalks were few and far between, limiting the kind of casual conversation you might strike up with a stranger while waiting at a bus stop or taking a walk around the block. That explains why I welcomed the driver of a delivery van bearing the logo of a local dry cleaner when he rang my doorbell one July morning.

"Good morning, ma'am. I'm Tom, of Westwood Dry Cleaning. I see you're new to the neighborhood and was wondering if you'd be interested in signing up for our free delivery service."

"It's a possibility. Let me talk it over with my husband."

"Sure. By the way, are you Jewish?"

Ouch! We had only been in the house about a month and already the anti-Semites were showing up on our doorstep? I decided to play it cool although I felt my *kishkes* (gut) tightening up as he reached his hand inside his jacket. Was there a gun in his pocket or was he really happy to see me?

Trying to maintain my equanimity, I coolly replied, "Yes. Why do you ask?"

Smiling winningly, he pulled out a business card from the pocket of his uniform jacket and handed it to me.

"I have a customer over on the other side of town. Mrs. Feldman? She's president of the local Hadassah chapter. Always asking me to be on the lookout for Jewish women who are new to the area. Her name and number are on the back of my card. She'd love to invite you to their next meeting. Can I give her your name?"

I had to stifle my urge to giggle at the absurdity of what had just transpired. "Of course you can. Thanks so much for stopping by."

"My pleasure. And I do hope you will consider becoming a customer." He cast a sly look in the direction of my abdomen. "You know, with a little one on the way, our low-cost diaper service would be a big help." And with a jaunty wave, he was off.

Turning the card over in my hand, I walked straight to the kitchen and dialed the number, unaware that thanks to Tom's welcome wagon visit that morning, I was destined to meet a woman who would become a lifelong friend until her death from brain cancer in 2021. May her memory be for a blessing.

Chapter 18

Girl, Interrupted

Song: "Nobody Knows the Trouble I've Seen" sung by
Louis Armstrong

The slide into sadness was a gradual one—until it wasn't. Like stepping into a lake and walking tentatively to find a spot in which you can begin swimming when suddenly, there is a deep drop off and you find yourself underwater, struggling to get back on top.

My initial step occurred when Melanie was three and a half. Having always been a sound sleeper, I began to have trouble falling asleep. If I did manage to get some shut-eye, I felt a sense of dread when I awoke, wondering how I would make it through the day and counting the hours until it ended. I gradually had less and less interest in eating, reading, theater-going, getting my hair styled, and sex. Activities that had previously provided pleasure now seemed overwhelming to even think about. I was always praying the next day would be the "turn card" one, but as time passed, I ceased to have hope for hope.

Years later, after Robin Williams's death, I began Googling

other comedians who had struggled with depression and found a plethora of names. Some were familiar like Jonathan Winters, Tig Notaro, Jim Carrey, Maria Bamford. Others I'd never heard of, the most unknown being Gary Gulman. His book *The Great Depresh* was about the debilitating course of depression that required hospitalization and electroconvulsive therapy (ECT). That was followed by *Misfit* in which he detailed being six months into his marriage when "a sinister third wheel in the form of crippling 'depression and anxiety' derailed his life and career," resulting in a move back to his mother's house.

Before I knew it, I was caught up in the nefarious addiction of web surfing, clicking on related links about other talented people who had experienced depression and/or committed suicide. Sadly, there was a wealth of information at my fingertips. I was drawn to those who had made their marks in the field of literature, as they wrote so intimately and eloquently about their struggles with mental illness in ways I could only have hoped to emulate: *Darkness Visible: A Memoir of Madness* by William Styron, the award-winning author of *Sophie's Choice*, and *The Noonday Demon: An Atlas of Depression* by Andrew Sullivan, a former editor of *The New Republic*, to name a few.

Clinical psychologist Kay Redfield Jamison's writings examine the link between mental illness and creativity, including her critically acclaimed biography of the poet Robert Lowell subtitled *Setting the River on Fire*. Dr. Jamison also authored other works about the topic, but she first came to my attention after I read a review of her memoir, *An Unquiet Mind: A Memoir of Moods and Madness*. Early in her career, Dr. Jamison chose to concentrate on bipolar disorder; later, in an ironic twist of fate, she was diagnosed as having the very same illness. In one of the most poignant passages, she writes:

"Others imply that they know what it is like to be depressed because they have gone through a divorce, lost a job, or broken up with someone. But these experiences carry with them feelings. Depression, instead, is flat, hollow, and unendurable."

One of the reviewer's comments especially resonated with me:

"Jamison makes it clear that she believes only those who have lived with clinical depression might know the implications of despair. Depression has nothing to do with emotions, it is an enduring pain that sucks all meaning out of existence. It affects all aspects of daily life."

Clearly, it was impacting mine and, by extension, my husband's. At his urging, in the spring of 1975 I began seeing a therapist weekly. The sessions were somewhat helpful in that I now had someone other than my husband to bear the brunt of my unhappiness, making his life less stressful. I upped the visits to twice a week but the more I unburdened myself, the more difficulty I had carrying out my responsibilities as a wife and mother. I felt as if I was simply an outline of myself, like a chalk figure of a victim at the scene of a crime—delineated as distinct from my surroundings with nothing but a void existing within the white lines. Yet the pain that emanated from that empty space was indescribable—literally. I was at a loss for words to express what I was experiencing because it was unlike any other feeling I'd had up to that point in my life. I had to struggle to maintain a sense of normalcy in the presence of others, especially Melanie.

One afternoon in late spring of 1976, I decided to take her to Van Saun County Park, a local recreation area that had a petting zoo, a train ride, and other attractions I thought would keep her entertained without making any major demands on me. Walking back to our car to head home, I felt disconnected from the world. A sense of heaviness pervaded my limbs, and a feeling of dread overcame me.

As if in a fog, I buckled her into her car seat while a minor tremble of anxiety rumbled through me. Minor because I was glad I had survived another day without doing any bodily harm to myself or my daughter but disconcerting because I knew another day would dawn in less than twelve hours, and the cycle would begin anew. Rinse, spin, dry, repeat.

Similar incidents began happening with increasing frequency. The one that presaged my first hospitalization took place on a Friday afternoon four weeks later. I had agreed to host a last-minute play date at the request of my friend Anita, who'd received an unanticipated callback for a job interview the night before. She too was having a difficult time being a first-time mother, as her family lived five hours away, her husband was emotionally abusive, and she had left a high-salaried job and promising career at IBM to be a stay-at-home mom. Anita was the only one of my friends I had confided in about my situation and she had been very empathetic. (Years later, Anita divorced her husband, moved to California to become a therapist, and now has a very successful practice in Los Angeles.)

Since Anita had been such a good friend, I wanted to repay her for her kindness. I agreed to watch her daughter for the two hours she expected to be gone. When she got back, I opened the door still wearing the bathrobe and slippers I'd had on when she left. I was visibly distraught, on the verge of tears. She quickly steered me back inside, sat me down on the couch, and went to phone Larry.

After what seemed like an eternity but was probably less than three minutes, she walked back into the den, put her arms around me and, in a sotto voce delivery to avoid having our kids over-hear her, said, "Larry is leaving work early to come home. I assured him I will stay with you until he gets here. We'll order in pizza for the girls and play Candy Land. Don't worry, everything will get straightened out." Anita was right. But neither she

nor I could have known at that moment that my life would take many more twists and turns before it would once again follow a straight path.

Chapter 19

It's Electric

Song: "The Electric Slide" sung by Marcia Griffiths

Englewood Hospital was the only in-patient facility where Dr. Burton, my psychiatrist, had attending privileges as her practice was primarily office-based. When I called her that Friday evening, she told me it would be best for me to go there first thing in the morning. I was relieved to hear this directive. At least there I would feel safe and secure, locked away from the outside world, absolved of all responsibilities other than to succumb to the ministrations and medications ordered for me.

After being processed through the admitting office, I was taken upstairs by one of the aides to the psych ward, which had less charm and cheer than the nearby DMV office. Oddly enough, I felt right at home because the drab institutional walls, dull linoleum floors, and unflattering fluorescent lighting reflected exactly how I felt. The aide escorted me to my room and immediately proceeded to go through my handbag and small suitcase in search of any potential self-harming possessions: sweatpants with drawstring waists, belts, pencils, tweezers, and other "weapons of mass destruction."

She introduced me to my roommate, a dark-haired woman who appeared to be in her late thirties, dressed in a lovely pastel-colored top and matching slacks, both of which hung like deflated wind socks on her bony frame. This was my first encounter with anorexia nervosa. By the end of my stay at Englewood, I had become well acquainted with the behavioral hallmarks of this disease as well as several others described in the *Diagnostic and Statistical Manual* (DSM), the bible of mental illness that gets updated periodically, each new iteration denoted by a Roman numeral.

I was there only one week. Other than some group therapy sessions, a few appointments with the staff psychiatrist, numerous clay ashtrays and mosaic trivets, daily doses of antidepressant medication and a new appreciation for daytime soap operas, I felt I had nothing much to show for my inpatient stay. When I saw Dr. Burton for my first post-hospital visit, she reassured me that the medicine would take some time to work before it kicked in.

I methodically marked off days on the calendar, charting my emotions and thoughts during each one, as the hospital's recreational therapist had suggested during her one and only visit to the ward. By day seventeen, the resulting graph didn't exhibit much variation from day one. I got increasingly nervous as the start of the new school year approached, knowing there were several back-to-preschool tasks that I needed to get done for Melanie. With Labor Day looming ahead, I spiraled back down to the way I'd felt six weeks earlier. I turned down invitations to holiday barbecues, picnics, and concerts, preferring to cocoon inside and wallow in my misery. It was becoming clear that my short hospital stay and the prescribed course of psychotropic pills had not worked the wonders I had been hoping for.

Next thing I knew, I was headed "over the river (the Hudson) and through the woods" (of Central Park) to the Upper East Side of Manhattan. Dr. Burton had referred me to Dr. Jessup, one of her New York City colleagues, because she felt I needed an "upgrade" from a community hospital to an academic medical center. Dr. Jessup was on the staff of Mount Sinai Hospital, the very same place where Melanie had entered the world four years earlier. This time, however, I was not in a hurry to get admitted, knowing full well that my length of stay was sure to be longer than that of my previous psychiatric hospitalization and the treatment more intensive. And while both of these predictions turned out to be true, they didn't result in significant improvement. This conundrum continued to haunt me after my discharge at the end of September.

Melanie's fourth birthday was less than ten days away and thankfully I managed to pull together a small celebration. My parents drove out from Brooklyn to attend. Over coffee and Carvel ice cream cake, they expressed concern about my lack of progress and casually let drop that the doctor who successfully treated my mother's earliest bouts of depression was still in practice.

"Why not schedule a consultation with Dr. Brody?" my father asked.

"He's in Brooklyn. Even without traffic, I'd be facing a three-hour round trip."

"Well, you can stay overnight with us."

With a "can't hurt, could help" shrug, I acquiesced.

I liked Dr. Brody the minute I met him. Unlike the other doctors I'd seen before, he was sincere but straightforward and had great compassion for my situation. He truly got what life was like for individuals with drug-resistant depression and offered a last resort treatment modality for those desperately seeking an alternative. If I were to capture his words in a song lyric, it would go something like this:

    (sung to "Jet Song," from *West Side Story* by Leonard Bernstein)

When you're depressed
You feel less than sublime
The victim of some
Metaphysical crime

When you're depressed
People don't understand
They yell and they tell you
Snap out of it, man

You would if you could
They're the ones with madness
You can't just snap out of
Malignant sadness

When you're depressed
You're messed up in your brain
You worry like crazy
'bout just keeping sane.

Asked if you sleep, eat,
Or want to make love
You check off the box
Labeled "none of above."

Your teeth go unbrushed
You stay in your pajamas

Won't return calls
Even the Dalai Lama's!

I've got a plan
And I think you should try it
It won't involve meds
Or a gluten–free diet
Shockingly simple
But not so the fee
It uses electricity.

By the end of the consultation, I had given consent to undergo a course of outpatient ECT (commonly referred to as shock therapy) to be administered over approximately eight weeks. I'd need someone to drive me home following each session and since my father had recently retired, he agreed to be my chauffeur. We fell into a routine of doing something pleasant afterward, like going for a walk, stopping off for ice cream sodas (something he did with my mom after her treatments), or taking in the latest movie. With each excursion, I allowed myself to feel slightly hopeful that the veil of unhappiness would begin to recede but approaching the end of December, I was fearful that it would still be hanging over my head after the last strains of "Auld Lang Syne" had faded away on New Year's Eve.

The first movie Dad and I went to see in January was *Camelot* with Vanessa Redgrave and Richard Harris. As the lights dimmed and the overture began, I felt a slight shiver of excitement. It sounds clichéd but the music struck a chord. I knew practically the entire score by heart because of the reams of Mr. Dupont's sheet music from that and other hit Broadway shows nestled in the piano bench at home. At some point, I found myself singing along with the soundtrack, my feet tapping in rhythm to numbers like "I Wonder What the King Is Doing Tonight." As we emerged out of the darkened theater into the sunlight, I realized for the first time in what seemed like forever, I didn't want the day to end.

Chapter 20

The Comeback Kid

Song: "Rise Up" sung by Andra Day

The current from the ECT not only shocked me back to health, it also jolted me into taking stock of my life and coming to grips with the fact that I was not content with being just a wife and mother. Feeling a debt of gratitude to Dr. Brody for making that happen, I considered resuming my original goal of becoming a physician. But how would I go about it without having all the necessary prerequisites?

Once again, my sister came to the rescue. By now Susan was a high school history teacher and one of her colleagues was the school librarian. She did some research and informed my sister that the School of General Studies at Columbia University had a post-baccalaureate program with evening classes for so-called "nontraditional students."

Fall semester 1977. I enrolled in Biology and General Inorganic Chemistry, even though I received an A in the latter when I took it at UB. The program had a statute of limitations on some courses if taken too long ago. The following year I took Organic Chemistry and Physics. Organic is notorious for being the premed class that separates the wheat from the chaff when it comes to getting into med school. It's academia's equivalent of the Hogwarts sorting hat in the Harry Potter series and it left me struggling to master the curriculum.

To my chagrin, I got a D on the first exam—a first in all the years I had been a student. I doubled down on my studying efforts and managed to inch up to a C minus by the date of the final exam, which would cover everything we'd been taught from day one. I calculated I would need to ace it just to be able to eke out a final grade of C. When the grades were posted, I was stunned. Next to my name was an A.

This fortuitous turn of events was because the professor had a very different take on grading students than his colleagues. Rather than weight each exam and compute the mathematical average of the resulting percentages, he assessed a student's overall progress during the semester. An A on the final proved to him that you had mastered everything he set out to teach for the semester. To this day, I am convinced that if not for that professor's enlightened grading system, I probably would not have gotten into medical school.

My physics professor was more old-school so I knew I would have to work my ass off in his class just to earn a B. Physics was my least favorite course in high school. What little I retained from Mr. Marantz's class I had all but forgotten a decade later. So, I had a lot riding on the two-hour final that was scheduled for 10:00 a.m. on an August day that was recorded as one of the hottest of the summer.

Being a stickler for punctuality, I allotted a good hour and a half for what was ordinarily a fifty-minute trip, traffic permitting. I was barreling along making good time until traffic came to a complete standstill midway across the George Washington Bridge.

I willed myself to remain unfazed, praying it was probably just an everyday fender bender and cars would start moving before long. *Wrong*! After about fifteen minutes, a news update came over the radio. "There's been a collision on the George Washington Bridge involving a tractor trailer hauling chickens from out of state. Better off taking the Lincoln or Holland Tunnel into the city as traffic is expected to be tied up for at least another hour."

Damn! The adrenaline started pumping, shattering all attempts to remain calm in the face of what I was convinced would result in academic catastrophe. Finally, cars in front of me began to inch ahead. Once I made it to the exit for Riverside Drive, the normal traffic pattern resumed. By the time I parked my car and raced across campus to Havemayer Hall, my watch read 11:25 a.m. Panic-stricken, I rushed into the classroom convinced the professor would not allow me to sit for the exam because of the lateness of the hour.

Thankfully, he had somehow gotten wind of the "fowl" back-up. (Sorry, couldn't resist). With a rueful smile, he motioned for me to take a seat. "Relax. I heard about what happened on the GW. You'll still have the allotted two hours to take the test." Thankful, I finished on time and earned a B minus in the course. Coupled with the strong grades I had earned up to that point, I entered the fall 1978 semester with a competitive GPA and began the medical school application process.

Unlike most of my younger classmates, I could apply only to a limited number of schools given Larry's occupation. He needed to be within commuting distance to the diamond district located in midtown Manhattan. The choices boiled down to Albert Einstein College of Medicine, New York Medical College (NYMC) and the two NJ state schools. Luckily, I was granted interviews at all four.

The closest school to my home was NJMS in the heart of Newark, site of the deadly eponymous riots in the summer of 1967. One of the precipitating factors was thought to have been a contentious 1966 "eminent domain" proposal to relocate the medical school from its original site in Jersey City to its present location in Newark's Central Ward, a move that would have forced the neighborhood's mostly black and Puerto Rican population to lose their homes. The end result was the establishment of the 1968 Newark Agreements that incorporated affirmative action hiring plans as well as a pledge to "assist the school in actively recruiting minority students, faculty, and professional staff."

Ten years later, signs of that turbulent time were still evident as I drove to the NJMS campus for the interview. It looked as if some sort of urban defoliation had befallen the area, reducing it to rubble-strewn, vacant grass-covered lots—an inner-city ghost town. I was relieved when I finally arrived at the university's fenced-in, outdoor parking lot adjacent to the entrance of the medical school. I took the escalator to the second floor which housed the Office of Admissions and Student Affairs. "Take a seat. Dr. Tesori will be with you shortly," the receptionist remarked offhandedly.

There was no shortage of chairs, as I was the only person there besides her. I found this surprising. At the previous interviews, there had always been at least a handful of applicants waiting to be seen. We'd usually be given a student-led tour, creating a camaraderie that helped allay some of our apprehensions and put us more at ease. This time, I was on my own. After what seemed like an interminable waiting period, the receptionist announced with a wave of her hand, "Dr. Tesori will see you now."

Dr. Tesori's title was Associate Dean for Admissions and Student Affairs, but he looked more like an absent-minded professor.

He was casually dressed in a nondescript shirt and pair of slacks, both of which would have benefitted from some time spent on an ironing board. He sported a black eye patch over one eye, making him seem more like a wannabe pirate than a distinguished dean. (Later on, I was told he'd lost sight in that eye due to cancer.) He proved to be a lovely, down-to-earth man and since there was no other applicant waiting to be interviewed, we had an unhurried conversation. I left hoping I had won him over. However, I would have welcomed the opportunity to see more of the school than just his office and meet enrolled students in order to get more of a "feel" for the school.

My final interview was at NYMC and there the experience was the complete opposite. For starters, the campus was in bucolic Valhalla, New York on a prerevolutionary site known as Grasslands Reservation. Westchester County purchased Grasslands in 1915 and subsequently constructed buildings that were devoted to the care of individuals with diseases prevalent at that time. One such structure was Sunshine Cottage.

The NYMC website contained a summary of its history. Built in 1931 as a thirty-five-bed children's tuberculosis hospital, its decorative motifs "symbolized health and happiness, and referred to the typical treatment regimen of rest, fresh air, and sunshine. The fanciful animals in the surrounding fences, the motifs of the rising sun and nature scenes over the windows and on the pediments, the rabbit over the door, and the animal sculptures that formerly resided on the pillars of the fences were designed to brighten the lives and speed the recovery of sick children."

The Admissions Office was now housed in Sunshine Cottage, which still retained all those fanciful period details. Getting there, however, required a winding drive past a modern-day addition to the Reservation—Westchester County Department of Correction. Encircled by a barbed wire fence, its stark architecture stood in marked contrast to the row of NYMC administrative buildings directly across the road, each reminiscent of modest English stone houses gone slightly to seed.

Understandably, the glossy NYMC brochure I'd received along with my interview invitation made no mention of the fact that a medium-security prison was located on the same premises as the medical school. Nor did it mention that students doing third- and fourth-year clinical rotations at the adjacent teaching hospital were sometimes called upon to treat prisoners. In the early years of the AIDS epidemic, many prisoners would be admitted in need of medical attention for complications from the newly identified disease; I was one of those students in my fourth year during an elective in hematology. But I'm getting ahead of myself.

The room where I was instructed to report was one of the two large lecture halls used to teach the first- and second-year basic science courses. It was nearly filled with applicants, all wearing the standard interview attire—wing-tipped shoes or preppy loafers with conservative, dark- hued suits and ties for the men; low-heeled leather or suede pumps and prim bow-tied blouses underneath unadorned black, navy blue, or gray suits for the women. The year was 1979 so my recollections of fashion norms are categorized by the standard "either/or" taxonomy of the times. As far as I know, terms such as "cis-male," "cis-female," "gender-fluid," and "nonbinary" had not even been coined when I was applying to medical school.

What was standard was a category on the application labeled "Sex." That never made sense to me because in my mind, sex was something you had or did not have, a distinction favored by Bill

Clinton as we learned during his impeachment. Years later, my hunch was confirmed when Diane Sawyer interviewed Caitlyn Jenner on national television about her dating preferences as a transgendered woman. When asked to clarify the difference between sex and gender, the Olympic champion assigned male at birth succinctly replied: "Sex is who you go to bed with; gender is who you wake up as."

There were several individuals standing in the front of the lecture hall clad in the unisex student uniform of jeans, T-shirts, and sneakers. These were the volunteer tour guides. They divided the applicants into small groups and showed us the library, student lounge, cafeteria, and lastly, the gross anatomy lab, while good-naturedly answering our questions and trying to allay our fears of what came next—an individual interview with a faculty member of the Admissions Committee.

I was dispatched to the office of Dr. Tucci, a short, dapper, dark-haired urologist with a genial disposition. He didn't lob any curve-ball questions my way or present any medical cases to challenge my scientific acumen. He seemed genuinely interested in my nontraditional premed trajectory and my extracurricular activity at a local community center's weekly "swim-in" for patients with multiple sclerosis.

On my drive back to New Jersey, I weighed the pros and cons of all four schools. The two in New Jersey had the lowest tuition as they were both state schools and easily accessible via the Garden State Parkway but some of their teaching hospitals would require long commutes. Albert Einstein was the most research-oriented but was in the Bronx and the Cross Bronx Expressway was notorious for big trucks and terrible traffic jams. NYMC was the costliest but had a beautiful campus and more diverse clinical affiliations including two city hospitals where students were known to receive extensive hands-on training and an opportunity to see patients presenting with symptoms of rare diseases such as leprosy. And if the very positive vibe I got from having spent two hours there was any indication, it was most likely the best fit for me. As I headed over the Tappan Zee Bridge and saw the Hudson River glinting in the Saturday afternoon sunlight, I realized that would be the best route for me to follow over the next four years in pursuit of a medical degree.

So, on February 14, 1979, I was thrilled when the mailman rang my doorbell at noon and handed me a registered letter welcoming me to the NYMC Class of 1983. Best Valentine's Day ever!

Chapter 21

Abracadavers

Song: "Can't Help Falling in Love" sung by Elvis Presley

I loved med school from the very first day. I will never forget the opening lines of my anatomy professor's lecture on reproduction: "We are born between urine and feces; or as you med school youngsters might put it, 'We play between pee and poop.'"

Larry sure didn't think we were playing very much during the first few weeks. "You spend more time bending over your cadaver than me. And when you finally do get home, you reek of 'eau de formaldehyde,' not exactly a scent conducive to cuddling."

I guess I did go a bit overboard with studying at the start. But I was overwhelmed. Our first assignment was to master the brachial plexus, an intricate complex of nerves emanating from the spinal cord that carries motor and sensory signals to the arms and hands. Dr. Dossett, the imposing European-born anatomist in charge of Gross Lab, was a stickler for experiential rather than book learning. Our class of 180 was divided into groups of four, each assigned its own cadaver, and she expected us to show up, scalpel in hand, for each and every lab session. But even a perfect attendance record was no guarantee you could master everything in the syllabus. So, it was not unusual to find students burning the midnight oil on weekends and holidays.

Luckily, I got some very wise advice from my college room-mate Bonnie's husband, Scott, the director of a residency training program in family medicine.

"Joan, you can't possibly learn everything, so don't even try. Concentrate on what's of primary importance. Think of it this way: don't study for your exams, study for your patients."

His words helped calm my nerves as my lab partners and I steadily dissected the nerves of our cadaver, as well as the arteries and veins traversing the musculature of her upper extremity.

Before we knew it, the first major challenge of our medical careers presented itself—the dreaded lab practical. "It vill be one week from today," announced Dr. Dossett in her European-sound-ing accent. "You vill need to know not only all the bones but the origin and insertion of all the muscles as well as names and func-tion of the nerves making up the brachial plexus. De Gross Lab will remain open over the weekend if you wish to 'bone up' on your ca-daver. Ha ha! But it is verboten to remove the skeletons from their closets unless someone from the lab staff is on site. Delmore, my assistant, he vill be on call in my absence. He is the only one besides me with the closet keys but do not contact him unless there is an emergency."

Dr. Dossett walked over to one of two steel lockers, unlocked it, and pointed to the pelvic area of the skeleton hanging from the top of it. "Zo, vat do you think this poor woman died from?" She paused a beat before exclaiming, "Vaiting for Mr. Right," and guf-fawed at her joke. The class, alas, did not.

Clearly disappointed by our lackluster reaction, she returned to her formidable composure. "I repeat, do not remove the skeletons from the closet. In previous years, students made off with the skeletons and took dem back to their dorm rooms to play silly pranks. So, now ve bolt dem in the closet like dis—jawohl, no more *abracadaver*." This time the class emitted forced laughter to placate her. It seemed to work. "Ha, ha. Dis joke, you find funny. *Sehr gut.* Any questions? *Nein?* OK, *auf wiedersehen*."

Delmore, the lab assistant, was a lot more easygoing. A perpetually smiling gentleman with an upbeat Jamaican lilt in his voice, he'd been a fixture at NYMC for many years and went out of his way to help stressed-out freshmen jump through the initial hoops of the first semester. When we complained we couldn't make out squat by peering into a dark locker in a dimly lit basement lab, he reassured us, "Don't worry, be happy. Who said anyting 'bout detaching it? You need to tink outside de box." He then lifted up the top of the locker revealing the skeleton was attached to it and shared his tips for passing gross anatomy in a reggae-inflected cadence:

Take de skeleton out of de closet
And bring it over here
Don't you worry about
Old Dr. Dossett
She not be one to fear.

You gotta master
Skeletal anatomy
Way down here in dis
Windowless academy
So, take de skeleton out of de closet.

Go hang it up
Right next to de drawing
Naming each body part
Den we'll get your
Imagination soaring
As Delmore demonstrates…
And free associates
De art of getting smart.

Dis here is de scapula
It be shaped like de cape of Dracula
A cape gets draped
Around de blades of your shoulder
The shoulder blade's de scapula
Like she told ya.

Learning medicine
Is not rocket science
It does take memorizing
And self-reliance
And wid free associatin'
You will get an "A."

Thanks to Delmore, I did. This gave me the much-needed boost of confidence that I could compete with classmates almost ten years younger, many of whom had graduated from Ivy League colleges and had already been named co-authors on peer-reviewed research papers. As the only female parent in the Class of 1983, I couldn't devote as much time to my studies as they did or fully participate in extracurricular activities. I did participate in the annual NYMC Follies, a student variety show written and produced by the second-year class at the end of spring semester, best described as *Saturday Night Live* crossed with *The Capitol Steps*.

I wrote and performed a parody of "Freddy, My Love," a doo-wop song from *Grease* sung by Marty, one of the Pink Ladies. In it, she declares her undying love and devotion for her boyfriend despite the distance and challenges that separate them. In my version, a nerdy first-year med student professes her unrequited love for her less than devoted boyfriend who turns out to be—well see if you can guess from the first verse:

Freddy, my love
I'm seeing more of
You each day
(ooh-ooh-ooh- ooh)
We're going steady
In a most peculiar way
(ah-ah-ah-ah)

Each day I'm by your side
From nine until fi-ive,
And our relationship
Continues to thri-ive
Yet you don't even seem
To know I'm ali-ive,
Freddy, my love, Freddy, my love
Freddy, my love, Freddy, my lo-ove!

Have you got it yet? If not, here's the bridge:

Your liver's all neurotic
Your lungs have got TB
There's just some plastic tubing
Where your colon used to be
The surgeon's fee got fatter
When he took out your gall bladder
And though I know you're a cadaver
Still your heart belongs to me.

I think I was fascinated by Gross Anatomy because I'd always been a visual learner. My nearly photographic memory enabled me to easily absorb and retain knowledge. This probably explains why Anatomical Pathology turned out to be one of my two favorite second-year courses. The other was Introduction to Clinical Sciences (ICS), in which we had our first exposure to patients. Once again, the class was divided into small groups and assigned to various NYMC-affiliated hospitals located in the five boroughs as well as Westchester County and Connecticut. My group was assigned to St. Vincent's Medical Center in the heart of Greenwich Village. It's no longer in existence but at the time was a large teaching hospital with many residency programs serving a diverse catchment area, making it an ideal place for students to learn how to take a medical history and perform a physical exam.

I would usually arrive early and grab lunch in the hospital's coffee shop. One afternoon, while I was eating with some members of my group, I looked up from my customary tuna-on-wholewheat to see Doreen, a Student Council officer, walking toward the table. She stopped in front of me and handed me an envelope with my name on it.

"What's this, Doreen?"

"It's a letter from Dr. Kikkawa." Dr. Kikkawa was the chair of the pathology department.

"Why would he be sending me a letter?"

She shrugged her shoulders. "I have no idea. But he asked me to deliver letters to a few others in the class as well. Sorry, can't stay and chat. I have Council business to discuss with the head of the med ed office in the other building. Gotta run."

I tore the envelope open and pulled out a single sheet of NYMC stationery. On it was a terse message instructing me to report to Dr. Kikkawa's office for a noon meeting the next day. I couldn't fathom what sort of transgression I had made to warrant a summons to the office of a department chair. My only consoling thought was whatever I'd done, there were others in the same boat.

My first instinct was to immediately call Dr. Kikkawa's secretary in order to see if she knew what the meeting was about. But the year being 1981—practically a prehistoric era for telecommunications since cell phones had yet to be perfected and available to the masses—this meant that I would run the risk of being late for class or missing it altogether in order to locate a pay phone, not to mention scrounging up enough change to use it. In the end, I shoved the letter back in its envelope, stuck it in my book bag, and headed off to class, a decision that most likely helped to save my life.

Chapter 22

Lumps and Bumps

Song: "Suspicious Minds" sung by Elvis Presley

"Today, you are going to learn how to palpate for lymph nodes," intoned Dr. Murphy, the preceptor for my ICS group. "These small, bean-shaped structures are part of the immune system. Hundreds of them are found throughout the body." He threw up a slide to illustrate this, accompanied by a quote from the American Cancer Society that he proceeded to read out loud.

"When there's a problem, such as infection, injury, or cancer, lymph nodes in that area may swell or enlarge to filter out the bad cells. Swollen lymph nodes, aka lymphadenopathy, tell you something is not right, but other symptoms help pinpoint the problems. For example, ear pain, fever, and enlarged lymph nodes near your ear are clues that you may have an ear infection or cold."

With a click of the projector switch, another slide popped up, this one depicting a close-up view of the mediastinum, the region between the lungs. "But as this shows, some lymph nodes lie deep within the body so that even if enlarged, they won't be palpable."

Dr. Murphy then turned off the projector, motioned for the

class to stand up, and announced, "We are now going to the bedside of a patient so that I can demonstrate the correct method of palpating for lymph nodes. Follow me." Obediently, my classmates and I donned our short white coats and trailed along behind him, looking like an entourage of white swans gliding dutifully behind their mother.

Once inside the patient's room, we fanned out around his bed to watch Dr. Murphy conduct his examination. He began by placing his hands on either side of the patient's lower face, and gently massaging the area adjacent to each earlobe in a circular pattern. Methodically, he worked his way down the patient's body, repeating this motion at various anatomic landmarks along the way. When done, he invited each of us to take turns replicating his palpations, offering course corrections when needed. At the conclusion of the exercise, Dr. Murphy thanked the patient for his cooperation, and we all traipsed back to his office to collect our belongings. "Next week, we will cover examination of the heart and lungs, so be sure to bring your stethoscopes. Class dismissed."

Ever the diligent student, that night after dinner I practiced what I'd learned earlier in the day on my own body. Imagine my surprise when my fingers detected a pea-sized lump in front of my left ear. I reassured myself that it was probably nothing to worry about as I felt perfectly fine. Nevertheless, I made a mental note to schedule an appointment with Dr. Cantor, the ENT specialist who had treated Melanie when she sustained an injury in the kitchen.

The next day I reported to Dr. Kikkawa's office a few minutes before noon. The secretary ushered me into the departmental conference room where a lovely buffet lunch was laid out. One by one, other students arrived until there were six of us seated around the table. None of us had a clue why we were there, but we speculated it couldn't be bad news if he'd gone to the trouble of providing lunch.

Precisely at noon, Dr. Kikkawa walked in and took a seat at the head of the table. He told us to help ourselves to the food and while we were eating, he enlightened us as to why we had been summoned to meet with him.

"I'd like to congratulate all of you on your excellent performance in my course. At this point in time, you are the top students in the class; if you continue to perform at this level, you will undoubtedly earn a final grade of honors. In light of your proficiency, I'd like to encourage you all to pursue a career in pathology and consider doing your residency training in our program after graduation."

A collective sigh of relief could be heard throughout the room. Dr. Kikkawa went on to tell us about the program and practically offered a position on the spot if we were interested. Of course, we were all very flattered but equally as naive because as second-year students, we knew very little about graduate medical education and the relative competitiveness of each specialty when it came to getting accepted for residencies. Compared to fields such as orthopedics, dermatology, and surgery, pathology was way down on the totem pole. As a result, many of the spots in pathology residency programs wound up being filled by graduates of foreign medical schools. Consequently, American medical students were often wooed to apply to their own school's pathology program before the residency application process had even begun. This was what Dr. Kikkawa had in mind all along when he'd asked us to meet with him.

Wow, I thought as I left the meeting to get to my last class of the afternoon. Life in medical school was turning out to be a bowl of cherries—except for that pesky lump that seemed to have popped up out of nowhere.

When I was done for the day, I phoned Dr. Cantor's office and asked for the earliest available appointment. Luckily, he had a cancellation for the following week. After examining me, he said, "I'd like you to see a radiologist. You might have Sjögren's disease." I remembered reading about this immune system disorder in which the body attacks the cells that make tears and saliva. "One of the common symptoms is swollen salivary glands, often the set located behind your jaw and in front of your ears. So, let's get a sialogram. It's an X-ray of the glands and the ducts leading to them." He handed me a referral slip and I started to head out of the office, but he beckoned me back and retrieved the referral slip from my hand. "And while you're there," he added while scribbling something on it, "you might as well get a chest X-ray."

With final exams coming up soon, I was tempted to postpone the referral. After all, I felt fine so what was the hurry? Common sense prevailed, and I took the earliest appointment. After the radiology technician completed both procedures, she told me to return to the waiting room while the radiologist read the films. I waited only a short while before the radiologist called me into his office.

"Please, have a seat. The good news is the sialogram is normal." He paused a minute to let me savor this information. "But it appears that you have a large mass in your mediastinum that needs to be followed up."

The first thought that came to mind was, *what a fine kettle of fish this is.* By the time I saw Dr. Cantor for my follow-up appointment, faint red blotches had blossomed on my forehead, more lumps and bumps had sprouted up, and it felt as if I had a lump in my throat whenever I swallowed. You did not have to be an honors student to realize this turn of events, coupled with the abnormal chest X-ray, warranted a biopsy. What I didn't know was that it would mark the start of a new chapter in my life, one in which I would get to experience pathology up close and personal.

Chapter 23

Two Years

Song: "Time (Clock of the Heart)" sung by Culture Club

"**I got the biopsy results** back from the pathology lab."

Last week of June 1981. Four days earlier, I had been admitted to the community hospital where Dr. Cantor performed biopsies from some of the suspicious lesions that had materialized since I first discovered the lump in front of my ear. I could tell by the downward slant of his lips and the droop of his shoulders that the next sentence was one he'd hoped he would never have to utter to a previously healthy, thirty-two-year-old wife and mother halfway through medical school.

"I'm afraid you have stage 4 non-Hodgkin's lymphoma."

He was afraid? I was terrified. Don't get me wrong—I had already steeled myself for a diagnosis of cancer. But since less than a month had elapsed from that fateful day at St. Vincent's, I had managed to convince myself that early detection had been instrumental in keeping any malignancy that had set up shop in my body from becoming a matter of life or death. The numeral that followed the stage of the malignancy was a game-changer, but I couldn't stop myself from asking the obvious question. "What's my prognosis?"

"Two years."

The same number of years it would take for me to graduate medical school. Oddly enough, this mental calculation offered me some solace in accepting my fate. I had worked so long and so hard to get into medical school, I wasn't about to give up now, even if it meant my degree might be awarded posthumously. I unclenched my fists, took a deep breath, and asked, "So where do we go from here?"

He gave me a very literal answer. "You need to transfer to a university medical center as soon as possible for a more thorough work-up followed by an aggressive course of chemotherapy."

Since I had given birth at Mount Sinai and my gynecologist was married to my husband's cousin, I turned to him for help in pulling some strings. I was admitted to the Internal Medicine service there just prior to the start of the July Fourth holiday and was informed my oncologist would be a doctor by the name of Yves Marcelin.

In my mind I envisioned Dr. Marcelin to be a handsome, suave, charming Frenchman with the kindly disposition of Maurice Chevalier in *Gigi*. While he did turn out to be a good-looking, well-dressed Parisian, his curt, aloof, almost condescending personality did not make for a very comforting bedside manner. If *Oklahoma!*'s Rogers and Hammerstein instead of *Gigi*'s creators, Lerner and Loewe, had written a scene and song depicting Dr. Marcelin's initial, no-nonsense explanation of my medical situation, here's what it might have sounded like:

DR. MARCELIN:

(seated behind his desk peering at a medical chart)
Oh, Lymphoma!
It's an oncological disease
You get lumps and bumps
Your fever jumps
And your T cells do just what they please

Oh, Lymphoma!
It's a cancer that's inclined to spread
To your liver, spleen
Points in between
And in two years you could wird up dead.

But we'll treat you definitively
With some heavy-duty chemotherapy

And you'll go bald
Your spouse will be appalled
But with a wig you could look just like
Dolly Parton
Even startin' today
How would you like to pay?
Mastercard is OK!

JOAN:

My husband is worried sick about me. Can you please talk to him and answer some of his questions?

DR. MARCELIN:

(stands abruptly)

Sorry can't help you with that

I've no time to sit around here and chat

I've got to go

I've rounds to make you know

I'll see you back here

Two days from now

For your work-up

Try to perk up,

Somehow

(sneaks a peek at his Rolex watch)

Mon Dieu, I can't delay

Au revoir, s'il vous plaît

Dr. Marcelin's persona was emulated by the medical team under his tutelage. As any devoted fan of *Grey's Anatomy* knows, patients in teaching hospitals are cared for by teams consisting of an attending physician, several residents, and one or two medical students. Each morning, they make rounds on the patients assigned to them, with one member of the team designated to update the others on what has transpired over the past twenty-four hours. Patient load and time constraints often don't allow for much in the way of introductory pleasantries with each patient. Sometimes, they aren't even acknowledged by name.

This was the paradigm that Dr. Marcelin had established for his team, as I found out when they rounded on me for the first time. A swarm of white-coated individuals filed into my room and fanned themselves out around my bed. The chief resident brandished his clipboard in front of him. Without even glancing in my direction, he intoned, "This is a new admission—stage 4, NHL. Chart says her prognosis is grim—two years at best. Spencer, please enlighten us as to the standard drug regimen for her condition."

Spencer was a third-year student. Internal medicine was his first clinical rotation. Once students reach this undergraduate medical education milestone, their lives are governed by the academic calendar of the hospital, which runs from July 1-June 30. This means Spencer had been a team member for less than a week. But he proved up to the challenge. Cheekily he replied, "A tasty, toxic cocktail of CHOP—cytoxan, hydroxy adriamycin, oncovin, and prednisone. She's due for her first 'sip' today."

The resident gave a smile of satisfaction. "Impressive for a newbie. I'll leave you to start her IV."

Suddenly, Spencer's smug smile turns into a nervous frown. "But I've never done that before."

"Well, you know what they say—see one, do one, teach one. Get going STAT. And when you're done, grab me a Danish and a cup of coffee. Not the crappy stuff from the cafeteria. Go to the Starbucks on Madison and Ninety-Seventh. Then meet me down the hall—by then we'll be with the gallbladder in room 217." He turned to exit, the rest of the team, minus Spencer, in tow.

On my bed tray, Spencer assembled the items needed to insert an intravenous line. He gingerly started palpating my forearm. Screwing up his courage, he slid the needle into what he hoped was a vein. "What a prick!" I exclaimed.

"I know. He's the nastiest resident at Sinai. Just my luck to get assigned to him."

"No, I mean the jab you just gave me. That hurt something fierce. I think you just went through my vein." Jokingly, I teased him, "I'll probably die from the puncture wound before the cancer does me in."

Hastily he withdrew the needle and apologized. "Gosh, I am so sorry. This is my first week on this rotation; I just started third year."

"Yeah, me too."

Spencer looked up in surprise as he removed the needle. "Oh, I didn't know you were a med student."

"Actually, in my school, we have the summer off between second and third year, so my first clinical clerkship doesn't begin until September. I'll be starting in pediatrics."

This news caught him off guard. "You mean you plan to stay in school?"

"Hell, it's taken me so long to get this far, I'm not about to drop out now."

"But according to what's written in your chart, you're scheduled to get chemo every three weeks for the next two years."

"So, I've been told. But I already spoke with my dean of student affairs who was very understanding. Before the start of each clerkship, he's going to notify the coordinator that I might need to take some time off during the rotation. And if it exceeds what's normally allowed, he will juggle my schedule so I that I can make it up."

Spencer nodded his head approvingly. "You're lucky he's willing to go to bat for you. I can't imagine the student affairs dean at Mount Sinai Med would ever be so supportive. Compared to him, Attila the Hun is a pussycat."

Now it was my turn to be taken aback. During my first two years at NYMC, I had never stepped foot in the dean's office as I never needed any help managing my affairs. I had just assumed that if I ever ran into difficulty, Dr. Robert Goldstein seemed like the sort of administrator who could be counted on for help. Spencer's words made me realize that I was indeed fortunate to have Dr. Goldstein in my corner as I rounded the bend toward the second half of medical school. The impact he made on me during those last two years lingered long after he handed me my diploma.

Chapter 24

Living on Borrowed Time

Song: "Do You Really Want to Hurt Me" sung by Culture Club

Dr. Marcelin had decided to schedule my first round of chemotherapy for the day before my discharge from Mount Sinai. As the time drew near, I was filled with both anxiety and anticipation. I was nervous about the litany of side effects I might experience from the four-drug regimen but eager to begin ASAP so that I would have ample time to recover from them before starting my first clerkship—Pediatrics—right after Labor Day.

A resident showed up late in the afternoon to start the infusion. Unlike Spencer, she managed to find a vein on the first try–so far, so good. I settled back in bed, mesmerized by the slow but steady *drip-drip* of fluid trickling from the bag on the IV pole into my arm. I visualized each spherical droplet as a Pac-Man avatar, traveling through my body to gobble up the villainous cancer cells threatening to kill me. So entranced was I by this imagery, I drifted off to sleep, only to be rudely awakened after what seemed like only an hour by an intense, overwhelming nausea unlike anything that I had ever experienced before.

Dragging the IV pole behind me, I stumbled out of bed and made it to the bathroom just in time for my GI system to erupt like Mount Vesuvius all over the bathroom floor. I had two more eruptions. When I felt there was nothing more to bring up, I gingerly got to my feet, cleaned myself off, and stumbled back to bed. The cycle repeated itself over the next twenty-four hours until finally, it came to an end and my trips to the bathroom ceased. I congratulated myself on having survived my initiation into the world of chemotherapy, a grotesque galaxy I was scheduled to inhabit for the next two years.

Luckily, I had been assigned to do Pediatrics at Metropolitan Hospital, a city health care center near Mount Sinai. To fit my chemo sessions into my academic schedule without taking too much time off, Dr. Goldstein suggested that I do them on Friday afternoons. He granted me permission to leave school early on the appointed days to make the half-mile walk across town in time for my appointment. This arrangement worked quite well. I would check into the chemo floor by 2:00 p.m. and with luck, pull into my driveway around 5:00 p.m.

When I got home, I placed a plastic-lined wastebasket next to my bed so that I could puke my guts out without ever getting up to go to the bathroom. On Sunday morning, I emerged from my chemo cocoon, ready to resume my studying for the upcoming week. To celebrate the return of my appetite, Larry, Melanie, and I instituted a family ritual. It consisted of going to our local Charlie Brown's Steakhouse for Sunday dinner, where I wolfed down two slices of its delicious bread slathered in butter, indulged myself at the all-you-can-eat salad bar, and polished off a twelve-ounce steak and a baked sweet potato the size of a small boulder. (I have fond memories of those Sunday family outings and often get to relive them because those items constitute the favorite menu of my granddaughter Marissa, although she likes Peter Luger steak sauce with her sirloin while I prefer mine "neat." The food preferences of her brother Ryan, on the other hand, lean more toward burgers and French fries and to my knowledge, lettuce and tomatoes have never passed through his lips.)

None of my remaining third-year clerkships were located near Mount Sinai, but they were all within commuting distance of my home. This allowed me to maintain a shortened school week when necessary. With time, the interval between chemo sessions grew longer as the drugs began taking their toll on my white blood cell count, a common occurrence when undergoing chemotherapy. Therefore, I didn't need to take as much time off and had a bit more stamina.

This was especially beneficial when I did my rotation in Psychiatry at Westchester County Medical Center (WCMC), the school's main teaching hospital. The caseload was high and students were expected to have a great deal of one-on-one therapy interaction with their assigned patients, as well as attend the many rounds and group therapy sessions that were a daily part of life on a psych ward (as I well knew.) Most of my peers were uncomfortable in this setting, preferring the more procedure-driven, results-oriented outcomes they associated with the other four mandatory clerkships—Internal Medicine, General Surgery, Pediatrics and Obstetrics/Gynecology.

I strongly suspect that had the school's administration surveyed each class at the end of third year, Psychiatry would have been ranked as the least favorite subject. Many of my classmates confessed that they were content to just make a perfunctory effort to get through what they considered a necessary evil of their medical school experience. Me? I had a different attitude that stemmed from my firsthand experience dealing with mental illness. I empathized with my patients, understood their frustration and sense of hopelessness, their rebellion against the tedium and isolation of daily life on a locked ward, the long wait to gain permission to use the dilapidated hall pay phone, the long queue at the nurse's station for the distribution of daily meds, and the lackluster enthusiasm they exhibited in the occupational and recreational activities that were designed to be part of the healing process.

I did the best I could to treat them with compassion and respect and encourage them to share bits and pieces of the lives they had lived before their mental health had taken a nosedive, so that I could get to know them as people rather than patients. I thought that was the least I could do in view of my lowly status as a medical student. Apparently, my superiors thought otherwise, as reflected in the midterm evaluations submitted to Dr. Artunian, the psychiatrist who oversaw the clerkship.

"You've received very complimentary feedback on your performance from everyone on your team, all the way from your resident to the attending. Clearly, you have the makings of a psychiatrist. Have you ever considered becoming one? We would love to have you join our residency program."

If truth be told, I had been toying with the idea since I began my psych rotation but quickly rejected it out of hand. Rightly or wrongly, I feared that my family history coupled with a career in psychiatry would somehow make me more prone to having recurrences of my own bouts with the "noonday demon," a risk I was unwilling to take. I was too ashamed to admit this to Dr. Artunian, afraid it would undermine his opinion of me and have a negative effect on my final grade. It wasn't until several years later, when

I became a medical education administrator advising students in choosing a specialty, that I realized my professional life might have turned out differently had I been honest about my dilemma with Dr. Artunian that day.

Instead, I managed to muster a facsimile of a smile, and nodded my head from side to side in what I thought was a signal that I was deliberating whether to accept his offer. After a pregnant pause, I came up with what I thought was a reasonably valid response.

"Thank you so much for your vote of confidence. I am exceptionally flattered by your willingness to accept me into your program even though I am only halfway through this rotation. But so far, I only have two clerkships under my belt—Pediatrics and OB/GYN. I think it would be best to wait until after I've done Medicine and Surgery and a few electives before declaring a specialty. I'm sure you understand."

Dr. Artunian reached over to shake my hand. "Of course, Joan. That's an eminently sensible approach. But my door is always open to you should you decide to apply to our program. We don't often find US medical students who want to go into the specialty, so when a student like you comes to our attention in the third year, you can't blame us for wanting to recruit you."

And I didn't. But to paraphrase Groucho Marx, I didn't want to belong to a profession that wanted to have me as a member.

Chapter 25

To Be...

Song: "Stronger (What Doesn't Kill You)" sung by Kelly Clarkson

The finish line was in sight. I would cross it in a matter of minutes. Graduation day had arrived, and I had survived long enough to take part in it. Thankfully, despite the odds I was in remission from non-Hodgkin's lymphoma. As the commencement speaker pontificated about the challenges that awaited the Class of 1983, I found my mind wandering back to the events of the past year and a half.

I couldn't help but marvel that I was sitting under a huge white circus-like tent that had been erected in the middle of campus to accommodate some seven hundred guests of 180 soon-to-be MDs. Like each of them, I was clad from head to toe in full academic regalia—black gown, tasseled black beret—holding the green velvet hood that would soon be placed around my neck by none other than Dr. Goldstein in a ceremony dating back to Europe in the twelfth century. Most of them had never set foot in his office so being hooded by him did not have the same significance as it did for me.

If he hadn't been so kind and understanding when I walked into his office unannounced on a cold, windy February afternoon in 1982, I would not have been walking up to shake his hand on this sultry Monday in the first week of June. Midway during my twelve-week clerkship in Internal Medicine at Lenox Hill Hospital, I had turned thirty-three. It was my first rotation at a large, private academic medical center. I soon began to feel overwhelmed by the rigorous daily routine, intense atmosphere, and severity of illness of my assigned patients, many of whom were in the advanced stages of cancer. I thought that hosting a Sunday birthday brunch for a few close friends might lift my spirits—which it did until the last guest departed and it was time to clean up. The task sapped the little energy I had left, leaving me too spent to thoroughly enjoy the rest of the day with my husband and daughter.

I went to bed feeling very guilty and continued to be preoccupied as I rounded with my team the next morning. With each successive patient report, I found myself thinking more and more about the toll that med school and my health were taking on my family. On my lunch break, I paid a visit to Dr. Goldstein to seek his advice. He suggested that I rearrange the rest of my third year by taking a one-month leave of absence followed by two electives and finishing Internal Medicine at a smaller suburban hospital in Connecticut. I did a quick mental calculation and discovered an unsettling flaw in his proposal.

"Won't that leave me one month short of completing the required number of fourth-year electives?"

"Yes," he replied in his customary unruffled manner. "But you can get a waiver of the requirement so that you can graduate on time."

Nervously, I asked, "Who do I have to see to request it?"

He reached across his desk, patted my hand, and said, "You're seeing him right now."

This scenario replayed itself in my head as my name was called, and I walked toward the stage to receive my diploma. Heading up the stairs, I heard NYMC's president announce that I was the recipient of the Board of Trustees award, given annually to a graduating student who, through inner strength and determination had succeeded in meeting and overcoming unusually difficult and testing challenges in the course of earning a medical degree.

The announcement was met with a thunderous standing ovation from my classmates, bringing tears to my eyes. When I reached Dr. Goldstein, I gave him my hood and bent slightly so he could drape it over my shoulders. After he handed me my diploma, I gave him a big hug, thinking that would be my last encounter with him. But Larry, bless his heart, threw me a surprise graduation party two days later to which he had invited Dr. Goldstein and his wife. Of all the presents I received that night his presence was the most meaningful.

Another surprise arrived about one week later, but this one was most unwelcome—a small lump in my left armpit. I knew it would need to be biopsied but between getting my daughter ready to leave for sleepaway camp and fulfilling all the preemployment requirements for starting my residency on July 1, I didn't have very much spare time. When I finally got around to calling the surgeon's office, the earliest appointment I could get was about a month away. I put it on my calendar and out of mind so I could finish sewing labels on my daughter's camp uniforms and attend the graduate medical education orientation for incoming residents.

It was not surprising that I decided on Pathology as my specialty. However, when and where the decision was made might seem somewhat unorthodox. It was the first elective I did upon return from my third-year leave of absence, and I chose to do it at WCMC. I had been a big fan of the TV show *Quincy, M.E.*, starring Jack Klugman as a forensic pathologist, so the fact that WCMC housed the county medical examiner's office made it an ideal place to be.

Given the center's proximity to the Hudson River, many of the autopsy cases that I observed were "floaters"—floating corpses. Though dead bodies initially sink, the gasses produced by postmortem putrefaction cause them to rise to the surface. The resulting stench is awful, as is their appearance, but the pathologist who I was shadowing put things in perspective with her opening remarks.

"Think of an autopsy as the patient's final physical exam. Accord the body on a slab in the morgue with the same respect and reverence you would a patient on the examining table or in a hospital bed."

The flip side of this noble sentiment is the flip aphorism: internists know everything and do nothing; surgeons know nothing and do everything; pathologists know everything and do everything but too late.

I have always been a visual learner, which is why gross anatomy and pathology had been my favorite basic science courses and how I managed to ace them. Plus specializing in pathology seemed more compatible with my roles as wife and mother as the working hours were a little less grueling than the more clinically oriented fields. Thus, it seemed the most sensible option at the time.

As with applying to medical school, geographical constraints governed where I could do residency training, limiting me to northern New Jersey or NYC. The best NJ program nearest my Bergen

County home was St. Barnabas Hospital in Livingston. But it required its residents to work on Saturdays, and I wanted to have as much time on the weekends as possible to spend with my family. Of all the NYC institutions that I considered, Lenox Hill was the closest to my husband's office, which meant I would be able to commute to work with him. It was also affiliated with NYMC, and I liked the idea of maintaining ties with my alma mater since I had fond memories of my time there. The program director was a refined gentleman who ran the residency with a velvet-gloved hand rather than an iron fist, unlike most of his counterparts at the other programs where I interviewed.

The very first day, each of the first-year residents was assigned to work up a case and present it to the department at the end of the following week. I cringed when I heard this news because I knew Larry had been looking forward to going away over the July Fourth weekend. I also knew I would feel compelled to work nonstop on my case presentation until the due date, no easy task since I would need time off for my biopsy, which was scheduled around the same time. Naturally, he was very disappointed when I told him I wouldn't be able to accompany him on vacation, knowing that it wouldn't be a very relaxing getaway for me if I went. I assured him I wouldn't mind if he went without me, so he made a reservation to go to golf camp in Vermont with his nephew.

I spent the weekend poring over slides in the path lab and reading journal articles in the hospital library to prepare for my presentation. It was a good distraction from thinking about my upcoming appointment with the surgeon. I thought the presentation went well. I didn't know the department chair had attended until I received a note from his secretary the next day asking me to see him. At the time I didn't really give it much thought. I just assumed it was standard operating procedure for him to give post-performance evaluations. But I wasn't prepared for how laudatory he was in his feedback.

"Dr. Liman, I was quite impressed with your case presentation. It was obvious you went above and beyond the specified requirements, something I've rarely seen in first-year residents so early in their training. I look forward to following your progress through the program."

It doesn't take a mind reader to predict my reaction. Instead of walking out of his office on air, I had to concentrate on putting one foot in front of the other, nearly paralyzed from the feeling of déjà vu that overcame me. I was back in the throes of imposter syndrome, although this time the stakes were much higher. I was no longer a carefree student who could just sit back and bask in the praise; I was now an entry-level, salaried hospital employee with many responsibilities and my decisions would have real-life consequences—in some cases, life-and-death ones.

Just two weeks into my job, I had already set the bar at a higher-than-expected level for my future performance appraisals. I hadn't intentionally set out to do it. I just naturally assumed my fellow employees had the same work ethic and exacting standards that anyone admitted to a competitive training program in a prestigious NYC hospital would possess. It wasn't until years later when I was employed at NJMS that I learned otherwise. That's where I often heard students shoring up each other's egos before exams by nervously joking:

"What do you call the student who graduates last in the medical school class?" To which they would glibly answer in unison: "Doctor."

Now I would be expected to keep up my perfectionist pace for the rest of the four-year residency program, a regimen that would inevitably result in even greater shortchanging my daughter and my husband of valuable family time. Complicating the equation was the possibility I might not even live long enough to complete it, considering that in a matter of days, I would be checking in as a patient at a nearby hospital where my own fate would be determined by whatever pathologist was on duty when my biopsy specimen arrived in the lab.

Not to mention that a new and highly contagious disease dubbed AIDS (acquired immunodeficiency syndrome) had begun to dominate the medical landscape. By 1983, it had become a major source of morbidity and mortality especially among homosexuals due to the nature of its transmission. As the Upper East Side was home to a large segment of Manhattan's gay population, Lenox Hill had already had its fair share of AIDS patients, a number of whom developed non-Hodgkin's lymphoma, a not uncommon complication. Just my luck, I was assigned to assist with the autopsy of such an individual the first week on the job.

Caught up in this perfect storm of events, I began to question whether I should even stay in the program. And as crazy at it may seem, as the date of the biopsy procedure approached, I found myself hoping it would be positive for cancer. That way, I could gracefully resign for medical reasons, avoiding the scorn and shame that I thought would otherwise follow me for the rest of my life. With bated breath I awaited the result. When it came, I broke down—literally. In layman's terms, I had a nervous breakdown and wound up in the 'summa cum laude' category of residential psychiatric facilities—Silver Hill.

Chapter 26

…Or Not to Be

Song: "Look For The Silver Lining" sung by Chet Baker

I **arrived at Silver Hill** on a beautiful Sunday afternoon in early August, 1983, huddled in the fetal position in the back seat of our station wagon. As much as I had protested going, I was almost relieved when I arrived. It turned out that the biopsy was negative, leaving me feeling as if the proverbial rug had been pulled out from under me. When suicidal thoughts started percolating through my brain, I knew it was time to wake up and smell the coffee. To paraphrase a line from the movie *Crazy for You* (2013; producer, Jennifer Handorf; director, James Moran), *"Many diseases can kill you; many patients in the throes of depression, hope it will. "*

I realized I needed help but the thought of returning to the bleak inpatient psych ward at Mount Sinai was abhorrent. Silver Hill, on the other hand, resembled an upscale country estate. Its clientele included many dual diagnosis patients—individuals with drug addiction as well as mental illness. Over the years it has housed many prominent celebrities including Mariah Carey, Michael Jackson, Billy Joel, Nick Nolte, and Catherine Zeta-Jones.

Located on forty-two acres in bucolic New Canaan, Connecticut, it was founded in 1931 by psychiatrist John Millett. The grounds consist of manicured lawns, fragrant woods, and wildflower meadows, all crisscrossed with streams and ponds. Many patients say the beauty of the campus is an important element of the healing process. This was certainly the case for me.

Once it was determined I didn't need to be under 24-7 supervision, I was free to roam the premises in between the mandatory therapy sessions. The weather was conducive to taking long walks and stopping to rest on the stone bench in front of a lovely little chapel. It also made it easy to go to and from the indoor swimming pool in just a bathing suit and cover-up, a trek I made as often as I could. Swimming had always been one of my favorite activities.

It goes without saying (but I will tell you anyway) that the cost at a place like Silver Hill is not for the fainthearted. Since it's not considered a hospital, insurance may not always cover it. I am forever thankful that these factors did not hinder my admission. Nor did it seem to be an obstacle for most of the other patients, many of whom did have dual diagnoses.

During the time that I was there, I estimated the average age of that group hovered in the midtwenties. A lot of them were trust fund babies who shared similar pre-hospitalization lifestyles (shopping at Saks, partying at Studio 54, vacationing in Vail), none of which resembled mine. They formed their own clique, sat together at meals and after dinner, could usually be found hanging out in the lounge, listening to music or playing cards and board games such as Trivial Pursuit. If Silver Hill were a high school, this group would be considered the in crowd. I wasn't a part of it.

During the day, the lounge remained relatively empty because we were all required to stick to our assigned therapy schedules. But one afternoon, during some downtime between sessions, I heard the strains of classical music emanating from the hallway leading to the lounge and peeked my head in to investigate its source. At the piano (a Steinway baby grand, of course), sat a young woman about my age playing Rachmaninoff's Piano Concerto no. 2 by heart. I recognized her from occupational therapy and knew her name was Nancy but little else. She was a nurse at a university hospital in the city and had been admitted to Silver Hill after an aborted suicide attempt. Thanks to our mutual interests in music and medicine, and our shared history of depression, we became friends. To this day, whenever I hear that piano concerto, I smile and think of her.

In addition to the psychiatrists and psychologists who were the mainstays of the hospital staff, social workers also met with patients to learn more about their family background and what role it played in their illness. At my initial meeting with Janet Humphries, M.S.W., I was given the task of drawing a detailed family tree using an asterisk to denote which of my relatives, if any, had a history of mental illness. Although my artistic skills are negligible, it was obvious from my crude sketch that while the Rubenfeld branch appeared well trimmed, the Goodman side of my family could have benefitted from some pruning. Rather than reproduce it here, I thought it would make more of an impact if I provided an aural equivalent, using the same piece of classical music—"Dance of the Hours" from the opera, *La Gioconda*— that Allan Sherman co-opted for his brilliant song parody, "Hello, Muddah, Hello Fadduh." If you know the melody, feel free to sing along.

Here's dad's father
That's his mother
And there's Paul, his

Younger brother
Dad's two sisters,
Baby Murray
But my father's side
Was not the cause for worry

Grandpa Gershon
Was a mild man
Not a strong-willed-
Type-of-guy man
Said to be
Ex-tremely nervous
His condition kept him
Out of wartime service.

Family tree
The linkage runs
Maternally
Genetics has been
Mean to me
I need to climb on down
And let my feet
Hit firmer ground

That's mom's sister
Dorothea
But for her,
No panacea
Was around when
She was aching

From great highs and lows,
Both so debilitating

My aunt Dottie
She was once wed
To a dentist
Name of Alfred
Had a baby
Couldn't raise her
Cause aunt "Dotty"
She got crazier and crazier.

Family tree
Had mental instability
Inherited by poor ol' me
Oh lordie,
Won't you help
Me climb
Out of this twisted tree.

Yes the Goodman
Family's gene pool
Had still waters
That ran quite cruel

To create me
Sperm and ova
Backstroked through them
In a tortured bossa nova

Joan Liman, MD

Chromosomal rearrangement
Helped give rise to
My derangement
But the lesson
I've learned from it
Is with proper help
I'll work to overcome it!

And I did. I went over my family tree with my psychiatrist, Dr. Kellner, sharing whatever I could remember about the asterisked relatives. Since I never knew Gershon, my mother's father, I had no firsthand knowledge of his mental health issues. But I got to witness Aunt Dottie up close and personal. She lived in a single-room-occupancy hotel in Manhattan that had seen better times in previous years, the kind where lost souls on welfare found refuge during the 1970s and 1980s. She was a tall, thin woman who was always garbed in ill-fitting black clothing from head to toe and carried a beat-up pocketbook the size of a duffel bag, the better to salvage discarded items she came across on the sidewalk that she deemed worth recycling.

Every once in a while, Aunt Dottie would take the subway from the Upper West Side to Brooklyn to have dinner with us. In addition to getting a home-cooked meal, she also received some money, thanks to the largesse of my father. The evening would start off well enough but inevitably something would set her off and she would begin ranting and acting erratically. Eventually, she would storm off into the night, screaming as she made her way back to the subway, her long black skirt flapping around her legs. All she needed was a broomstick and pointy hat and she could have been a doppelgänger for Margaret Hamilton as the Wicked Witch of the

West in *The Wizard of Oz*. (Years later, I conjured up this image of her when I tried out for the role in a community production of the show. Lo and behold, I got the part.)

I also told Ms. Humphries about my mother's mental health struggles. Although her mood swings were not as pronounced as Dottie's, they definitely made an impression on me and my sister. My sister often bore the brunt of them because she was more rebellious than me and would stand up to her. Seeing the fractious interchange between the two of them was unsettling for me, as were the bruise marks on my sister's arms. I took the opposite route and resolved to be the good little girl who would avoid doing anything to displease her out-of-control mother. As a result, I grew up determined to give my best to anything I undertook, and tended to take on more than I should, often at personal expense.

Upon hearing this revelation about my mother, Ms. Humphries nodded her head and gave me a wry smile. "Coming-of-age in the feminist movement spearheaded by Betty Friedan, Gloria Steinem, and other women's lib advocates in the late 1960s probably helped contribute to the continuation of your behavior into adulthood."

I shot her a quizzical look. "Not sure I follow your train of thought."

"Your generation of women grew up hearing the mantra, 'You can do anything you want or be anything you want.' But it didn't include an unsaid caveat. You can't do it all—and do it all well—at the same time."

True that! Her statement unraveled the inner turmoil I had been experiencing for the past two years while battling cancer. I felt I had to choose between my marriage and my medical career at a point in my life where I didn't know whether I'd even be alive to see my daughter reach puberty. I loved my husband and my daughter too much to take that risk. While Ms. Humphries was helpful in clarifying my dilemma, I was at a loss as to how best to resolve it until a conversation with a fellow patient provided the solution.

Anthony was a Yale University staff psychiatrist being treated for drug addiction.

"Why don't you consider being a doctor who doesn't doctor?" he suggested.

"Come again?"

"Just as there are plenty of corporate lawyers who suffer burnout from working eighty-plus hours a week and decide to use their legal degrees in less stressful ways, there are nonpracticing physicians who opt to put their medical education to use in health-related fields with less demands on their time and energies than the specialties for which they trained."

"Like what?"

"Pharmaceutical advertising, insurance firms, TV and newspaper reporting, drug companies to name a few. Plus, teaching and administrative positions in hospitals and medical schools."

My chat with Anthony was astonishingly therapeutic. It gave me a new outlook on life, so much so that after a month had ended—along with my insurance—I was pronounced well enough to be discharged. More importantly, it provided concrete advice that ultimately paved the way to a job that I hoped to hold until retirement. But as the saying goes, "Man plans and God laughs." Who knew God would prove to be such a stand-up comedian when it came to my life?

Chapter 27

School Daze

Song: "Be True to Your School" sung by The Beach Boys

"**D**r. Liman, Dr. Frost on line two."

"Thanks, Theresa, put him through."

Theresa was the secretary in the Office of Academic Affairs at UMDNJ. I began working there in the summer of 1992, nearly a decade after receiving my medical diploma. My first job after medical school was as assistant dean for clinical affairs in the NYC administrative office of Ross University. Ross was one of many proprietary "offshore" medical schools that had sprung up in English-speaking Caribbean countries in the 1970s, the best-known being St. George's University, School of Medicine in Grenada. If the name sounds familiar, it's because then President Reagan sent troops there in 1983 to protect US nationals, including students, from protests precipitated by the assassination of the island's left-leaning prime minister.

Ross is located in Dominica, whose terrain is lush, almost junglelike. As at the other offshore schools back then, its students typically spent two years studying basic sciences on campus, followed by two years studying clinical sciences in US or British hospitals.

That's where I came in. Once the students returned from Dominica, I was responsible for them. In order to help them make a smooth transition from their classrooms and labs on the island to the hospitals and clinics on the "mainland," one of my responsibilities required flying to Dominica each semester to conduct an orientation for the rising third-year students.

I know what you're thinking—it was a tough job, but somebody had to do it, right? Actually, the job itself was a no-brainer; better yet, my daughter and husband came along on the Caribbean jaunts enabling me to have a family vacation and work at the same time, an option that had never before been available to me. The real challenge was getting to the island as there were no direct flights from NY airports to Dominica, circa 1984. My preferred route was to fly nonstop to Antigua and transfer to LIAT airlines for the short hop to Rousseau, the island's capital. LIAT is the official acronym for Leeward Islands Air Transport. Most people joked that it really stood for a host of other, more colorful names. A 2013 article published in Britain's *Daily Mail* cited alternatives such as "Luggage Is Always Tardy," "Languishing in Airport Terminals," or "Leave Island Any Time." It also included a sarcastic letter written by a disgruntled passenger, claiming his luggage went lost during a "nightmare flight that stopped at six airports." The postscript? "Keep the bag...I never liked it anyway."

On my first trip, I was accompanied by a handful of my colleagues as the plane had a single-digit maximum capacity. It was a beautiful day with an awe-inspiring view of volcanic cliffs and black sand beaches as we made our descent. The only landmark that wasn't visible—at least to me—was the runway. Still no sight of one even as the pilot instructed us to put on our seat belts and prepare for landing. When I questioned my seatmate as to its whereabouts, she patted my clenched fist and calmly replied, "See that windsock? It's right there." She pointed to what looked like a Band-Aid that ran in front of a small, dilapidated building.

When we landed, someone came out, took our luggage off the plane (mine was lucky enough to have made it on board from Antigua), and motioned to follow him to the building that turned out to house both the customs and baggage areas, each accessible by separate doors. After having our passports screened and stamped, we exited "customs" and reentered next door to pick up our luggage. All the while, a cow stood grazing in an adjoining pasture, swatting flies and eyeing us dolefully.

On subsequent trips when my family joined me, I was able to squeeze in some sightseeing with them in between meeting with the students and faculty members. Many of the latter had held high-level positions at American and British universities and medical schools but decided to retire to the Caribbean where they could continue to work at a more relaxed pace and enjoy a lower cost of living in their golden years.

When the students returned to the US for their final two years, I rarely met with them or their instructors unless they had been assigned to hospitals in the New York metropolitan area. Since at that time, students from foreign medical schools were prohibited from doing more than twelve weeks of clerkships in the state of New York, they often traveled to places such as Florida, California, Illinois or in some cases to England to cobble together the number of clerkship weeks needed to graduate.

This decentralized paradigm of medical education had me shuffling a lot of paperwork and fielding a lot of phone calls rather than interacting with people. I left after a few years to seek a more fulfilling position. After two false starts, I landed a job in UMDNJ's

Office of Academic Affairs.

The office was located in Newark but had oversight for all the schools underneath the UMDNJ umbrella at that time. Consequently, I got to meet higher-level administrative personnel at the various and sundry meetings I attended on a regular basis, many of which were held at NJMS because of its proximity to this central office. It was at one such meeting that I met Donald Frost, a microbiologist who also served as senior associate dean for education at NJMS. We hit it off immediately, often going out to eat lunch or grabbing a post-meeting coffee in the school cafeteria. When a snowstorm turned into a blizzard during one workday, threatening to make my customary thirty-five-minute drive home via the Garden State Parkway a nightmare, he graciously invited me to stay overnight at his house, a ten-minute drive on local roads. That was my initial introduction to his wife, Kathy, who eventually became a close friend.

So, when Theresa told me Dr. Frost was on the line, I happily reached for the phone. "Hi Don, what's up?"

"Kathy and I are having some folks from the medical school over for a get-together this Sunday and we'd love for you and Larry to join us."

"Thanks so much. We'd love to come."

"Great. As long as I have you on the line, I wanted to ask you something. Did you know that Margaret Backus is planning to retire at the end of December?" Margaret had been the school's associate dean for student affairs for years, so this news didn't come as much of a surprise. "I was wondering if you knew of anyone who could replace her?"

His question caught me off guard. Was he asking because he genuinely wanted my input regarding potential candidates, or was he fishing to see if I would take the bait? I decided to bite. "How about me?" I tentatively replied.

"I was hoping you'd say that. Having seen how you've handled yourself in the past year and a half, I think the job will fit you like a glove. Why don't you start effective January 1 but spend a part of each day until then shadowing Margaret in the last couple of weeks she's still here? That way, you won't feel like a deer caught in the headlights on day one."

His prediction turned out to be right. The job was an ideal fit for my priorities—mental health, marriage, and motherhood—while putting my past education and achievements to good use. I used to joke that I was a Jewish mother to seven hundred students, "kvelling" over those who did well and nudging the ones who needed to do better as I shepherded each class from orientation to graduation.

Interestingly, there seemed to be a common denominator for both groups—almost everyone was on medication for one mental health issue or another—ADD, OCD, depression, social phobia, anorexia, test anxiety, you name it. Walking through the cafeteria, I would often hear them discussing their drug regimens as openly as they swapped details of their sex lives. Their conversation brought to mind the traditional Passover tune "Dayenu" ("Enough") and inspired me to compose this self-referential parody:

Chorus
Student #1 *I'm on Paxil*
Student #2 *I'm on Zoloft*
Student #3 *I'm on Prozac*

All
It acts to keep us sane. *Oyveynu!*
Student #1 *He's on Prozac*

Student #2 *She's on Paxil*
Student #3 *She's on Zoloft*

All
A sackful every day.

Verse (all)
Thank God now there's medication
Used for the eradication
Of anxiety, agoraphobia.

Side effects are oh so common
It says so here in this column
(they pull out medication insert pamphlets from the pockets
of their white coats)
Check the package insert for complete details.

Diarrhea, grand mal seizure
Muscle weakness and amnesia
That's perplexing, downright vexing
Gutten yu! (Translation: Oh Dear God)

Chorus (all)
A swell solution
Is this Wellbutrin
Celexa's also helpful
In cases such as these.
We'll keep trying
To keep from dying
If our ailments do not kill us

The very treatment will.
Oy!

As it was a state school, almost all the students were New Jersey residents. Compared to other US medical schools at the time, each class had a sizeable percentage of underrepresented minorities (URM), evidence of the school's commitment to the Newark Agreements and its dedication to affirmative action.

Since I had no role in the admissions process, I was unaware of any student's undergraduate credentials unless the individual had self-referred to my office or was mandated to report to me, most commonly for failure to meet the school's academic standards. At that point, I would read through the entire file in order to get a more holistic impression of the candidate than objective metrics such as grade point averages and MCAT scores alone could provide, especially since these were known to be more predictive of success in the basic science coursework of the first two years than the clinical science courses of the last. A few incidents that occurred early in my NJMS tenure are illustrative examples of this finding.

The first occurred a few days before orientation. Campus security called me to report a parking lot incident involving an incoming student with an Ivy League pedigree. Tracy had called their office to request a parking spot in the school's indoor garage, unaware that university policy required students to provide their Social Security numbers in order to secure one there. After the person on duty asked for hers, she became very hostile, angrily declaring that such a policy was not only an invasion of her privacy but illegal. When her abusive behavior continued unabated, he contacted me to report her.

Shortly afterward, Tracy called me to complain not only about the policy but his behavior. I explained that my office had no jurisdiction over campus security, nor could it make exemptions to official regulations but informed her that she would not be required to share her Social Security number if she parked in the outdoor lot that was open to the general public. The one caveat was that she should allow extra time to get to her first class because spaces there filled up quickly.

That was the last I heard of Tracy until her third year, as she had sailed through the basic sciences with flying colors. Once she began her clerkships, it was a different story. Her classmates and supervisors felt she wasn't a team player and were put off by her "prickly" demeanor. Her interactions with patients were similarly off-putting. Descriptors such as "haughty," "narcissistic," "imperious," "confrontational," and "demanding" peppered her clinical performance evaluations but high marks on the standardized written final exams saved her from ever failing a course. Nevertheless, she would show up in my office bemoaning why she wasn't "honoring" her clerkships as she had done in basic sciences, citing "personality differences" as the underlying reason for her subpar clinical performance.

Tracy's lack of insight was eye-opening to me. I suspected it was likely to continue unabated unless she sought professional counseling. To this day, I wonder what type of career trajectory Tracy the Ivy Leaguer had after she received her diploma.

The second one involved a senior, Louis, who was two months shy of graduation. Louis had applied to medical school during his senior year of college but was rejected, most likely because of his low grade point average. He got a job working in the IT sector but continued to harbor hopes of becoming a doctor so he enrolled in postgraduate science courses to improve his record. For the most part, his progress through NJMS was uneventful.

When a letter from what I gathered was his soon-to-be former wife ended up on my desk, stating that Louis should not receive his diploma, I was quite taken aback. She maintained that Louis had falsified his academic transcript the second time he applied to NJMS by using his computer expertise to alter some of his grades. After confirming her claim, the case was referred to our Student Honor Code Committee, chaired by a fellow senior. They recommended dismissal, an action that was upheld by the university's promotions committee. Instead of walking across the stage at commencement, Louis parted ways with the school one month shy of receiving his diploma.

The final and most egregious case didn't come to my attention until the individual was already in his residency but in retrospect, there may have been red flags even before he entered medical school. Like Louis, Brendon hadn't started medical school immediately after college. A divorced fireman with two children, he was already enrolled by the time I began working at NJMS so I never got to know him very well. I had heard rumors that he might have been involved in starting some of the fires that his unit had then been called to put out but to my knowledge, they were never substantiated.

Brendon's career goal was to become an orthopedic surgeon. While his grades were not stellar, his prior career was a plus and so he was able to obtain a residency spot in his chosen specialty at a nearby inner-city hospital. That was the last I heard of him until a few years later.

May 1999. I was in the kitchen making dinner and my husband was watching TV in the den. Suddenly, I heard him shouting excitedly, "Joan, Joan, get in here. One of your students is on TV."

When I got there, I saw a tall, muscular dark-haired man clad in an orange jumpsuit and sporting handcuffs as he was being "perp-walked" in front of a courthouse. He had been identified as a graduate of NJMS who had been arrested because he had tried to hire a hit man to kill the supervisor at the hospital where they both worked.

According to the next day's newspaper report, Brendon thought that his boss was writing negative job evaluations of him and was trying to hold back his career because of bad blood over a woman they had both dated. Earlier that month, Brendon had confided in a friend that he wanted to kill his supervisor and was looking to hire a hit man. Instead of calling a gangster, the friend contacted the authorities, "who arranged for an undercover investigator to meet Brendon in the parking lot of a sporting goods store not far from the hospital. When Brendon gave the investigator a down payment on a thirty-five-hundred-dollar contract, he was arrested on charges of conspiracy to commit murder and attempted murder." He ultimately went to prison.

These were just a few of the eye-opening moments I experienced while at NJMS. The others revolved around the qualitative differences in the academic backgrounds of many of the URM as compared to their non-URM counterparts. A number of them were first generation, first of their families to graduate high school, let alone college, and their secondary schools tended to be underfunded, understaffed, overcrowded, and offer fewer AP courses. Educational challenges like learning disabilities often went undetected until they reached medical school; even if they had been picked up earlier, their parents may not have had the time, knowledge, and/or resources to advocate for accommodations on their behalf.

On the other hand, there were non-URM students who had been diagnosed as having such academic challenges early on in their schooling but whose parents did not want to address them. Often, they declined to seek accommodations for their children, including drug therapy, for fear they would be stigmatized or labeled as different. In some cases, they removed their children from public schools and sent them to private ones where class sizes were small and specially trained educators were on staff to provide additional, individualized attention. Test preparation for standardized entrance exams like the SAT and ACT were often part of the standard school curriculum.

Socioeconomic factors played a role in compiling the non-scholastic components of an applicant's pathway to a career in medicine. Costly extracurricular activities (and parents with schedules flexible enough to chauffeur their children to them or the financial means to buy them a car), as well as unpaid volunteer work in a research lab that could result in a coauthorship on a paper in a prestigious medical journal, were worthwhile résumé-builders that could help compensate for lackluster test scores; however, they were luxuries beyond the reach of many individuals in our applicant pool. Their life experiences were often overlooked or underestimated, a regrettable oversight as they usually revealed personal characteristics indispensable for a profession that is an art as well as a science.

This dichotomy was the original impetus for the adoption of affirmative action in higher education. The idea was that by finally acknowledging the way the real world of higher education admissions worked, and instituting measures to level the playing field, we could promote equal opportunity. But in recent years there has been a spate of court cases challenging it. As reported by the American Civil Liberties Union (ACLU), a landmark June 2023 ruling by the US Supreme Court in the cases of Students for Fair Admissions v. Harvard and Students for Fair Admissions v. the University of North Carolina "overturned affirmative action in higher education, restricting universities' ability to fully address systemic racial inequalities that persist in higher education. This decision is the latest in the Supreme Court's move to break with decades of precedent and undo long-held civil rights."

Given this state of affairs, perhaps the time has come to explore an alternative pathway to ensure equal opportunity access to those seeking entrance into the profession of medicine albeit with the understanding that once admitted, they will be expected to demonstrate the requisite test-taking skills to pass the three-part standardized medical licensing exam (aka the boards), the first two of which are given during the second and fourth years of medical school.

Keep in mind that a diploma measures the ability to master a school curriculum; a license demonstrates the achievement of an *acceptable* level of competency to practice medicine. As Sir William Osler, known as the founder of modern medicine, observed: "Medicine is learned by the bedside, not in the classroom." Have you ever seen an undergraduate or medical school transcript displayed alongside a medical license in the offices of any of the doctors who you have visited? My guess is no.

On the other hand, framed copies of the certificates attesting to where they completed their residencies and fellowships almost always adorn the walls along with their medical school diplomas. Fred Epstein, MD, was found to have dyslexia as a child and struggled in school, leading his parents to wonder what would become of him. After graduating from NYMC in 1963, he trained at Montefiore Medical Center in the Bronx and NYU Medical Center. He went on to become a renowned pediatric neurosurgeon, responsible for developing groundbreaking procedures that helped children around the world.*

A potential mechanism that warrants serious consideration

for a course correction in admissions is a mandatory requirement for students to spend at least one year after high school in a national service corps. This idea has been put forth before, most notably in 2019 by Pete Buttigieg in his presidential campaign. To show my support for "Mayor Pete" and his proposal, I wrote a letter to the editor of *The Washington Post* that was published in a May 2019 edition. It was a recycled version of a 2017 unpublished op-ed piece I had submitted to *The New York Times* in response to an editorial by columnist Roger Corman. Several years later, I created a composite document to incorporate the most salient points of both, so that I could resurrect it when the time seemed right to send up another trial balloon about the idea. Unfortunately, with the 2024 presidential election only months away, there were more existential issues that warranted the public's attention. OK, time to get off my public soapbox and on with my personal saga…

When I was not seeing students on a one-on-one basis, my duties included serving on a myriad of committees, overseeing the selection process and induction ceremony for Alpha Omega Alpha (AOA), the national medical honor society, and running annual events such as the freshman White Coat Ceremony, Junior Year Residency Fair, and Senior Awards Day. I loved my job at NJMS so much that I used to jokingly remark to Don Frost, "I should pay the school to work here."

He, not so jokingly, replied, "Be careful what you wish for, Joan." With my career going well and my family still intact, I thought that my days of dodging lemons were finally behind me. Then my husband discovered yet another, considerably large one.

In the fall of 1998, we had bought a condo in Florida with the intention of becoming snowbirds upon retirement. Our first visit was in late December. While spooning in bed one night, Larry's arm brushed against my right breast. "What's this?" he asked, a distinct note of concern in his voice.

"What's what?" He took my left hand and guided it to the area in question. Still facing away from him, I palpated it. "Oh, it's probably nothing to worry about," I breezily replied. "I'll call my OB/GYN in the morning and make an appointment for the week we get home." It was a good thing that my back was still toward him. Despite my reassuring tone, the expression on my face was quite to the contrary.

Tragically, Dr. Epstein sustained a serious head injury in 2002 while bicycling and suffered a subdural hematoma. He died in 2006.

Chapter 28

Cancer, Act Two

Song: "Here You Come Again" sung by Dolly Parton

Let's cut to the chase. In January 1999, eighteen years of remission from non-Hodgkin's lymphoma, I was diagnosed with Stage 3 breast cancer and advised to undergo a mastectomy by Dr. Alisan Goldfarb, one of the preeminent breast cancer surgeons in New York City. I was devastated when she broke the news to me. At the same time, I couldn't help but appreciate its inherent irony. In the Jewish religion, each letter of the Hebrew alphabet has a corresponding numeral. The corresponding numerals of the letters in the word *chai* (life) add up to eighteen. At every happy occasion in the Jewish circle of life, joyous shouts of *l'chaim* (to life) permeate the air. Think back to scenes of Jewish births, weddings, and bar or bat mitzvahs in any movie, TV program, or theatrical presentation and you're sure to have heard this age-old toast. It's even the title of a showstopping number in one of the most iconic Broadway musicals of all time—*Fiddler on the Roof.*

Hearing Dr. Goldfarb proclaim, "You have cancer," after eighteen years of being cancer-free put a totally different spin on this number. Instead of a toast to long life, it now connoted possible death. Even more ironic was the fact that I was no stranger to breast surgery. Or to paraphrase Dr. Phil, it 'wouldn't be my first time at the surgical rodeo.'

"There goes Mount Everbreast." That's the charming moniker hurled at me by puerile males when I passed through the halls of Cunningham Junior High School. As if I were not self-conscious enough about my large breasts, another legacy of my mother. My ample-sized hips kept me from looking way out of proportion, but I still bought heavily underwired bras and hiked up the straps as far as they could go to contain their considerable heft, leaving deep, painful indentations in my shoulders. My posture was horrible because I constantly walked hunched over to conceal them as much as possible. And buying bathing suits? As one of those males might say, "Forgeddabout it!"

Hellish does not begin to describe that shopping expedition. Back then, purchasing a two-piece for big-busted teens like me was a bait and switch scenario. The tops did not come in cup sizes so I had three options: 1) go with a matronly one-piece that made me look like Grandma Moses; 2) purchase two two-pieces in different sizes or 3) surreptitiously switch the tops hoping I would not be caught in the act. (My apologies to any of the saleswomen at Abraham & Straus who had to explain to their managers why there were so many mismatched items in the swimwear department after I left their floor.)

Things literally went further downhill postpartum. My breasts hung nearly to my waist, one decidedly bigger and droopier than the other. I could no longer find department-store bras that fit and resorted to having them custom-made by a company called Edith Lances. The cost was prohibitive and there weren't any Victoria's

Secret-like styles to choose from.

So, after my first cancer diagnosis, I vowed if I made it to age forty, I would give myself a very special present. And I began shopping around by interviewing plastic surgeons. The one that came the most highly recommended was Dr. Michael Khanna. Allow me to indulge in some artistic license to portray how the consultation went down:

Me: Dr. Khanna, I want to be frank.

Dr. Khanna (puzzled): You want an operation to make you a man?

Me: No, but I would like to be less of a woman…

…I wanna get something off my chest
Can you please decrease the size of each breast.
I know that augmentation
Is the latest hot sensation
But I don't want more, I want less!

Dr. Khanna:

Most men I know would be oh so proud
To be wed to a gal so amply endowed.
May I ask your motivation
For this drastic renovation
Of the generous donation
Mother Nature's made to you?

Me:

I know it's kind of hard
For you to digest
With your masculine ideal

Of the female chest.
But I've thought about doing this
For quite some time
Here is why I've made up my mind:

I've got a constant ache
Across my back
It's starting to affect
My sacroiliac.
Lordosis, scoliosis
Are lying in wait
Because I'm too ashamed
To ever stand up straight.
My deltoids are hurtin'
From the strain of this burden
And my pecs—well they're
Strained beyond belief
Plus I'm tired of putting up
With catty locker-room grief…

Nurse: *(clearly intrigued)*
Boy, your boobs hang low
Wow, they wobble to and fro
Can you tie them in a knot
Can you tie them in a bow
Can you throw them over your shoulder
Like a continental soldier
…boy, your boobs hang low!

Dr. Khanna *(examining me):*

From your waist down to your feet
You're really quite petite
But my God your upper torso
Is its own Las Vegas floor show!

Me:
Believe me when I tell you
Fuller isn't finer
When you try to buy lingerie
From a fine designer
A racy, lacy teddy
Or a camisole
Just won't cover or contain me at all

If I'm to walk down the street
With my head held high
Shoulders drawn back
Nipples pointed to the sky
Dressed from head to toe
In Versace's best
Tell me Dr. Khanna—
Tell me are you gonna—
Help me get something
Off my chest.

And he did. About three pounds. As soon as I healed, I went on a wild shopping spree, luxuriating in buying a new wardrobe for my new size 34B figure, never dreaming in a million years that more downsizing lay in store.

Since there were no signs of cancer in my left breast, I didn't need or want a double mastectomy. But I did want reconstruction so Dr. Goldfarb referred me to a wonderful plastic surgeon. She outlined various options but the one she suggested was the TRAM flap, a relatively new technique in 1999.

"Why don't you go into the examining room, and I will explain it further. My nurse Grace here will escort you. Take off all your clothes and put on the paper gown that's on the table, opening to the front." Duh! "I'll be there in a minute."

I did as I was told and sat down on the examining table to wait for her. After a short while, she reentered bearing an anatomical model of the female torso. Pointing to the abdominal area, she matter-of-factly explained, "TRAM is short for the transverse rectus abdominus myocutaneous muscle. What I will do is use the skin, fat, and muscle from that location to make you a new breast. I will begin by separating a 'flap' of this tissue but not totally disconnecting it. Next, I will 'tunnel' it through the abdomen and up and out through the site of the mastectomy, where I will mold it so that it looks like your remaining breast as much as possible."

"What about a nipple?"

"Good question. After you've completely healed, which will take a few months, I'll have you come back to the office to create the areola and nipple out of the transplanted tissue. Then I will ink them with a color to closely match the shade of the nipple area on your remaining breast."

"You mean ink, as in 'tattoo?'"

"Exactly. Is that okay with you?"

Never in my wildest dreams did I think I would be 'packing ink' at the age of fifty. Now it sounded sexy!

"Sure. Let's go for it."

"Okay. Hop off the table, stand up straight, and lower the

gown."

After palpating my breasts and dictating some measurements to Grace, she put her hands on her waist, took a step backward, and studiously peered at the area below my waist. Shaking her head from side to side, she urged me, "You've got to let me do those hips."

I boldly retorted, "If you throw in the liposuction for free, it's a deal."

"Ah...no. But since I will essentially be removing most of your potbelly to create your new breast, you'll be getting a free tummy tuck."

"Deal."

On my way out of the office, I booked her first available surgery slot, February 1, 1999. As I was wheeled to the OR on the appointed day, I tried to distract myself by thinking about the fiftieth birthday party I had long ago decided to throw for myself if I survived NHL by the time I reached that milestone. Three months earlier, I had gone ahead and booked a venue, ordered invitations, and started dress-hunting, never dreaming that a second bout with cancer might derail it. As I was transferred from the gurney to the operating table, I looked up and saw the masked faces of my all-female surgical team—the breast surgeon, the plastic surgeon, and the anesthesiologist—peering down at me. The last thought I had before Dr. Shah inserted an IV into my arm was this: it's inconceivable that God is a female because what woman would have sat by and let me undergo elective breast reduction surgery at age forty—at considerable pain and out-of-pocket expense—only to need a medically necessary reduction covered by insurance ten years later?

Then I drifted off, confident this sisterhood of saviors would do its very best to prolong my life at least long enough to enjoy the fruits of my event-planning efforts.

Chapter 29

The Second Time Around

Song: "Hope for the Best (Expect the Worst)" sung by Mel Brooks

"Your surgery went very well, and you seem to be healing nicely."

It was my first post-op visit to Dr. Goldfarb and I was pleased she was pleased. Yet I was still on edge because I knew the operation was just the appetizer on the menu of a very long and laborious dinner party. Main course: several months of chemo with a side of side effects. Salad: a heaping serving of radiation (five days a week for six weeks). And for dessert—a dollop of an antiestrogen drug to be taken daily for the next five years.

"I'd like for you to start chemo as soon as possible."

"How soon is soon?"

"By the fifteenth of February."

"Is it possible we could postpone it until after the first Sunday in March?"

"Why is that?"

I told Dr. Goldfarb about the big bash that I had planned for myself on March 5 and how I was reluctant to cancel because of how much money would be lost on down payments. From the skeptical look on her face, I knew she needed more convincing. "Remember, I've been through chemo before, so I know how crappy it is. A joyous celebration surrounded by loving family and friends is just the kind of send-off I need before I begin round two. A sort of pre-procedure prep. Like cleansing your gut before a colonoscopy? Think of it as a morale booster to clear negative thoughts from my brain and lift my spirits, something to happily look back on when I'm cleaning the clumps and strands of hair from my bathtub drain or the foul-smelling vomit I spew all over my Laura Ashley comforter because I don't have time to even hunch over the edge of the bed and aim for the plastic-lined wastebasket I've placed there." I guess the graphic nature of the latter part of my off-the-cuff argument was enough to convince her.

Larry, on the other hand, was a harder nut to crack. He had good reason. The spouse or significant other of a person undergoing cancer treatment is a guest at that dinner party as well, if only vicariously. To be invited to partake in a second one had come as quite a shock. His sensitive nature, which was part of what I loved most about him, made it very difficult for him to deal with the slings and arrows of outrageous fortune that had befallen us. I tried to put myself in his shoes the best way I knew how—by composing a song from his point of view to reflect what was going through his mind the second time around:

> I've seen you wage this war before
> And though this time the enemy is different
> The rules of engagement remain unchanged
> Rules that make me feel so estranged
> 'Cause they place us in parallel worlds.

We dwell in parallel worlds
Barreling on past each other
Oh, it's hell, these parallel worlds
They keep us apart from one another.

You on the front lines
Like a modern Joan of Arc
Fighting to escape
Being burned at the stake
By the fiery flames of your illness.
While I remain all alone in the dark
Having the desire for you to quell my fire
But instead left to simmer in solitary stillness.

We dwell in parallel worlds
Barreling on past each other.
Damn, it's hell, these parallel worlds
And the feelings I can no longer smother.

I yearn for the days
When our lives intersected
And we lay connected
With our limbs entwined.

Now you spurn my advances
And my meaningful glances
You summarily dismiss as if
I'm out of my mind.

Joan Liman, MD

We dwell in parallel worlds
Where your priorities
Come before mine.
Me, well I'm expected
To just fall in line.

I'm left feeling helpless, out in the cold
While you're off to battle, fearless and bold
I know you're in a fight for your life
And you're trying to score a victory
But you don't seem to realize
The collateral damage
In the war that you're waging is...me.

Serious illness always takes a toll on those around us. But reliving this part of my life makes me realize just how tough things must have been for Larry during a large part of our marriage. He never bargained on having me go off to med school as Melanie went off to first grade, let alone having me bring my work home with me, so to speak.

And chemotherapy only added insult to injury because once again, I tried to schedule my sessions on Fridays so I would have the weekends to recuperate and be back at work on Monday mornings. I was AWOL from my duties as a wife and mother during that time frame.

Plus, I wasn't feeling particularly attractive or amorous thanks to the physical changes caused by the therapeutic poisons coursing through my veins. Not only did I lose the hair on my head; this time around, I lost it everywhere—eyebrows, lashes, even my pubic region. Nowadays, a naked va-jay-jay is considered the sine qua non of femininity. But in 2000, shaving one's nether region hadn't yet caught on. I felt more like a prepubescent teenager than a sexually mature woman. So, when the effects of chemo eventually wore off, allowing my vulva to regenerate the hirsute carpet that had once adorned it, I took it as a badge of honor. I returned to getting my legs and lips waxed on a regular basis but I steadfastly resisted the salon owner's pitch to purchase the "full spa package" with a pledge to remain the way nature had intended me to be:

I've got hair down there
And I don't intend to go bare
Every single molecule
Of every single "folli-cule"
Is gonna stay intact
Yes, that's a fact!

I've got hair…down there
And I don't intend to go bare
It's curly and coquettish
So, if you have a fetish
For baby-bottomed labia…(beat)
Go hump a camel in Arabia

Recalling that the amount of leisure time I had been able to spend with Larry during my first bout with cancer had been seriously diminished by the demands of mothering a preteen and making it through med school, I decided to try to keep up my stamina this time around because I didn't want him to resort to playing the cancer card if I begged off doing something he wanted to do. But he was less than enthusiastic when I told him that I wanted to go ahead with my birthday celebration.

I didn't realize just how much until a few days before the party when he came home from a round of golf and found me hunched over the dining room table. I was focused on doing the seating arrangement for the sixty or so guests I'd invited. Always wanting to add pizzazz to whatever event I orchestrated, the invitation specified the occasion would include a "roast and toast," so they could get up and say a few words if so inclined. I had also invited two of my musically talented NJMS students to perform a parody of Marilyn Monroe's famous paean to diamonds from *Gentlemen Prefer Blondes*. My title? "Discipline Is a Dean's Best Friend." But that afternoon in early March, my most important guest made it clear he did not approve of my party-planning efforts and intended to boycott the event.

"What are you doing—planning your own memorial service?" Larry incredulously exclaimed. "Soliciting eulogies? Choosing your own music? It's morbid and I don't want to be any part of it. So, don't expect me to show up." I realized his outburst stemmed from love rather than anger because he was afraid that this time around the malignancy merry-go-round, I might fall off and never get up. Nevertheless, his words struck a nerve, making me wonder whether subconsciously that had been my plan all along.

Even before my first bout with cancer, I'd always joked that I was such a control freak, I would probably want to stage my own funeral to ensure it would be a celebration of my life rather than a mournful homage to my demise. I had even toyed with the idea of composing a song encouraging mourners to donate to my favorite cause—supporting live theater—by purchasing a ticket to a show of their choice. But I wouldn't admit this to Larry, so I resigned myself to not having my plus-one at my side come the big day.

Being the mensch that he was, Larry did show up in the end.

That would have been a gift in and of itself. But he surprised me by walking up to the microphone after what I assumed would be the last speech of the evening to say a few words and hand me a gift. I had previously told him I wanted a dress watch for my birthday, and we had gone shopping to look for one a few weeks before. However, instead of the diamond-encrusted Ebel timepiece that we both admired, the box contained an unadorned Timex with a plain leather strap. By way of explanation, he announced to the partygoers that he specifically chose it because "like a Timex watch, Joan takes a licking and keeps on ticking."

That gesture reminded me of one of the many reasons why I had fallen in love with Larry in the first place—his values were in alignment with mine and he truly understood what was important to me. The fact that he was handsome and sexy as hell didn't hurt either. He received the standing ovation of the evening, and I couldn't have been prouder. (FYI—he did present me with the Ebel watch after we got home. Sadly, it went missing a few years later during one of our moves. But the Timex still sits prominently displayed in its original case on our fireplace mantel.)

Buoyed by the success of my fiftieth birthday bash, I was ready to face the rigors of chemo the following Friday. After six months, I segued into the next phase of treatment—daily doses of radiation for six weeks. The procedure itself took about ten minutes; the one-way commute to the hospital took thirty. I arranged to have the first appointment each day for two reasons: the machines often tended to break down as the day went on and I wanted to be at my desk as close to 9:00 a.m. as possible. This arrangement worked well. Though I became increasingly more fatigued after each session, I was still able to put in a full day's work throughout the entire course of treatment.

So far, so good…until I progressed to the third phase of the regimen in the fall of 1999: Tamoxifen, an oral antiestrogen drug that would be required for the next five years. After only a few weeks, I began to feel the familiar stirrings of depression coming over me, distracting me from performing at my usual level at work and at home. When I confided this to my oncologist, he reacted less worried than I would have expected.

"Oh, depression can be one of the side effects of Tamoxifen." *What the fuck*, I thought. It would have been nice if he had given me a heads-up about this, considering my past medical history. Thankfully, before I had time to work myself into a panic, he smiled reassuringly.

"Not to worry. We can switch to Arimidex, a commonly used alternative." He pulled out his prescription pad, scribbled something, and tore off the sheet of paper with the flourish of a knight in shining armor. "Unless you have any problems with it or concerns about anything else, I won't need to see you back here for another six months."

I felt like I had just been granted parole from a life sentence of misery. To me, the possibility of descending once again into the hell of mental illness was a fate worse than the pain of any physical disorder, even one as life-threatening as cancer. I know what you're thinking, "She really must be crazy." But hear me out. If I were a contestant in the final round of a TV game show hosted by God, and she/he/they (or any other personal pronoun preferred by that deity) posed the question, "Joan, over the years you had no choice about the various lemons I've lobbed your way. What if I were now to tell you that before you leave this Earth, you have to deal with one more…but this time I will give you a choice: cancer—anywhere in the body—or depression? For a thousand dollars, what's your answer?"

I would reply, "God, give me cancer and spare my mind." When a body part or organ is affected by illness, you can try to harness your brain to confront and cope with it. When your mind is the very entity that is being ravaged by a disease like depression, it is impossible to wrap your brain around anything else. It's as if you've been thrown into a torture chamber and you are both the torturer and the victim.

Fortunately, I haven't been faced with making such a Hobson's choice and hopefully never will, thanks to the advances in oncology and psychopharmacology that have transpired over the past twenty-plus years. In addition to switching cancer drugs, I switched to a different psychiatrist since mine had retired by then. After going over my chart and talking with me at length during my first visit, he made a most unusual pronouncement.

"I believe the correct diagnosis for the type of mental illness that you've had all these years is most likely bipolar disorder, type II." Huh? I didn't see that coming. "While all forms of bipolar disorder are characterized by shifts in mood and levels of activity, BPD II causes hypomania, a less severely elevated state than mania, and the episodes of depression outnumber those of mania."

"Why did I never learn this in medical school?"

"The term wasn't in use then. It was introduced around 1994 to help doctors describe and treat the condition more effectively."

"But if I had signs of mania, why didn't I or those close to me ever notice them?"

"Good question. Seems like an oxymoron, I know. In your case, it's probably because they weren't pathological." A smile escaped his lips. "They probably contributed to making you the optimistic, highly accomplished, very productive, extroverted, staccato- speaking woman I see sitting before me. Here, take a look at this." He opened his laptop to do a Google search, then swiveled the screen so I could read the results.

Because many of the symptoms of hypomania are often mistaken for high-functioning behavior or simply attributed to personality, patients are typically not aware of their hypomanic symptoms. In addition, many people with BP-II have periods of normal affect. As a result, when patients seek help, they are very often unable to provide their doctor with all the information needed for an accurate assessment; these individuals are often misdiagnosed with unipolar depression. BP-II is more common than BP-I, while BP-II and major depressive disorders have about the same rate of diagnosis. Of all the individuals initially diagnosed with major depressive disorder, between 40 percent and 50 percent will later be diagnosed with either BP-I or BP-II.

As more information has come to light about the disorder, there has been a call to end the distinction between types I and II. As with autism, the argument to be made for doing so is that it is more realistic to see bipolar disorder as a spectrum with a range of symptoms, patterns, and severities.

For nearly three decades I'd labored under a false impression. After reading the Google entry, I was left feeling I had been subject to a medical catfish scam by the psychiatric profession and was now due reparations. To paraphrase one of Linda Ronstadt's greatest hits, "I felt cheated, been mistreated, when will I be healed?"

"Will the change in my diagnosis affect my treatment going forward?"

"I want to tweak it just a bit. In addition to your current antidepressant, Paxil, I am going to prescribe 100 mg of Lamictal to be taken daily. Together, they ought to keep you on an even keel and protect against future episodes of depression or hypomania."

This change most likely explains why eighteen months later, when I got axed by the newly appointed dean, I didn't get depressed, I got mad—thanks to the effective medication keeping my breast cancer at bay, my new psychopharmaceutical armor, and my support group of colleagues with whom I shared my tale of woe. As befitting my thespian tendencies, I cast myself as a damsel in distress and the dean, a psychiatrist by training, as the villain. For the sake of anonymity and irony, I dubbed him Dr. "Dopa Mean," a mischievous example of word play since the actual spelling—dopamine—is the name of a substance that transfers information between neurons. Known as the "feel-good" neurotransmitter, it contributes to feelings of pleasure and satisfaction as part of the brain's reward system. The dean's action had exactly the opposite effect on me.

Formerly the dean of McMaster Medical School in Ontario, Canada, Dr. Dopa Mean had been recruited to NJMS in 2001 with a mandate to improve its bottom line. By that time, the corporatization of postsecondary education, including health professions schools and academic medical centers, was well underway. Students had become "customers," patients were rechristened "consumers" and deans were charged with becoming "rainmakers." The modern medical school dean was expected not just to oversee the training of future doctors and researchers but to raise the money to make it happen.

Although I'd seen Dr. Dopa Mean in passing we had never been formally introduced. That fateful April day in 2001, I thought I had been summoned to see him so shortly after he came on board so that he could congratulate me on having just won a Golden Apple award, commend me for being made an honorary member of the

NJMS Alumni Association, or compliment me on my crowd-pleasing gig at the Ottawa conference. Little did I realize how far off base I was. With apologies to Gilbert and Sullivan, here's my recollection of the scene in his office.

Time: 9:05 a.m.

Setting: A lavishly appointed conference room; oil paintings of NJMS former deans decorate all the walls with the exception of an empty space for the still-to-be completed portrait of Dean Dopa Mean. He is seated behind an ornate desk in a throne-like chair.

DEAN:

Come in, have a seat.

DR. LIMAN:

(enters)

It's nice to finally meet you.

(extends HER hand in greeting)

DEAN:

(ignores it)

Afraid I have some bad news for you. I'm asking you to step down from your position as of June 1. It's nothing personal. I just want to bring in my own person.

SONG

(to the tune of "I Am the Very Model of a Modern Major-General" from *The Pirates of Penzance*)

I am the major model of a modern major med school dean
Hired to economize and fire people sight unseen
Though trained well in psychiatry
Heartless I intend to be
If I am to administer
A leaner, meaner deanery.

DR. LIMAN

(in an aside to the audience)

I was mad as hell
Didn't take it very well
When told that he wanted to replace me
He claimed, "Nothing against you
It's a Canuck I once knew
So, here's your severance pay
Arrivederci!

To add further sodium chloride to the wound (I'm trying to stick to the medical imagery conceit here–just go with it), subsequently I found out he wasn't bringing on his own person. In fact, he was bringing on my own person—a part-time practicing NJMS physician whom I'd befriended, then mentored when she told me that she wanted to transition from clinical duties to a part-time administrative job. Think Bette Davis in the classic movie, *All About Eve*, after she finds out Anne Baxter, playing the ingenue, is gunning to replace her. However, I got to savor the sweet taste of schadenfreude a few years later upon hearing the Dean of Mean had so alienated the faculty after only a short time on the job that he'd been asked to leave, followed by my protégé soon after.

Yes, I'm taking some liberties in telling the tale of how I got downsized and deceived. That's because gallows humor has always been my fallback position when I'm faced with personal obstacles. The dean might as well have put a noose around my neck that day. Getting fired at the age of fifty-two from a job that I loved and hoped to retire from seemed like a death sentence. I felt like a victim of identity theft. Without a paycheck and a business card, I was stripped of the professional bookends I had always counted on to shore up my life. My job *was* my life! Eventually, I came to the realization that this setback was just one more loss I was meant to overcome, one more lemon to be squeezed in my "LimanAde Life."

But the anger was soon replaced by the anguish of the events that unfolded on September 11. Although I didn't know anyone who worked in the Twin Towers, the horror of what had taken place on that day consumed my thoughts, causing me to reexamine my personal and professional life, and contemplate a way to make both more fulfilling. I found myself thinking back to a radio interview that I had stumbled across one muggy Sunday afternoon shortly before the attacks. It stuck in my mind because in those days, I hadn't yet become a devotee of public radio as I am now. For some inexplicable reason, that day the dial was set to NYC's National Public Radio station. I got up to change it but stopped in my tracks when I heard an announcer say, "Today, we have with us the artistic producing director of New York City's renowned Amas Musical Theatre, Donna Trinkoff. Hello, Donna and welcome. Can you start by telling us the history of Amas and its mission?"

He had me at "Hello." I sat back down and listened as Donna began answering his question. "Amas, which is Latin for 'you love,' was founded in 1968 as a nonprofit, multiethnic theatrical organization by acclaimed actor Rosetta LeNoire and remains true to her vision of a color- and culture-blind theater company. It is devoted to the creation, development, and professional production of new American musicals, the celebration of cultural equity and minority perspectives, the emergence of new artistic talent, and the training and encouragement of underserved young people. It proudly celebrates its impact in pioneering multiethnic casting in the American theater and reiterates its commitment to this reflection of our diverse society. We are always looking for volunteers to help us carry out our mission."

How had I never heard of this organization? Me—a baby boomer who came of age during the civil rights movement and a devoted musical theater aficionado to boot? How fortuitous that I learned about it at a time in my life when I needed it most. Was it just random coincidence or was it what Carl Jung described as synchronicity—when two seemingly unrelated occurrences are attributed to somehow being linked although there is no causal connection between them. The cosmic intertwining of the two events was reinforced when I phoned Donna and told her that I had heard her NPR interview the day before and was responding to her call for volunteers.

After a long pause, she said, "What are you talking about? I wasn't on the radio yesterday. What you heard was a replay of a program NPR aired several years ago." Whether you chalk it up to synchronicity or the adage that coincidence is just God's way of staying anonymous, hearing her interview turned out to be a life-changer for me.

Chapter 30

There's No Business
Like Show Business

SONG: "I Wanna Be a Producer" sung by Matthew Broderick

"**Y**ou remind me of a friend. I think you should meet her. Her name is Virginia Criste."

Those three sentences were uttered in the spring of 2007 by Robb Hunt. He was the executive producer of the Village Theater in Issaquah, WA, a Seattle suburb. Robb made this suggestion toward the end of a brunch I was hosting in the garden of my midtown Manhattan pied-à-terre. I had donated it (the meal not the apartment) as a silent auction item for Theater Resources Unlimited (TRU), a group founded to assist individuals interested in becoming producers. In the aftermath of September 11, Larry's daily commute to his midtown office had become a nightmare and since I was unemployed, we decided to move to the city. By that time, Melanie had gotten married and vacated her studio apartment in Greenwich Village, so we took over her lease and moved in. When the lease was up, we purchased the one-bedroom garden apartment farther uptown that was within walking distance of Larry's office, the theater district, and Museum Mile. I took full advantage of the proximity to all three. There were often days when I went to MoMA (The Museum of Modern Art) in the morning, took in a Broadway matinee, and then met Larry for dinner.

Around the time the novelty of this new phase in my life began to wear thin, I received a phone call from a former NJMS colleague. He wanted to let me know that the New York College of Podiatric Medicine (NYCPM) was looking to fill the position of dean of students and admissions. I had planned on taking some downtime before beginning a job search but the opportunity to branch out into admissions was enticing. The school was in Harlem, four subway stops away on the Lexington Avenue line. I wouldn't need a car to get to work and I could continue volunteering at Amas, which I certainly intended to do. It seemed like a win-win situation all around. I applied for and got the job.

From the very beginning, the school's dean and I didn't see eye to eye about educational philosophy as it applied to podiatric school admissions and promotion standards. Suffice it to say I took a more rigid approach than he felt was warranted. Early on a Monday morning in mid-June 2002, after only nine months on the job, he summoned me to his office. When I saw the head of Human Resources already seated in front of him as I entered, I had a feeling of déjà vu.

"Dr. Liman, after thoughtful consideration, we think it's best that we let you go." Saddened but not surprised, I nodded my head in rueful agreement. "When will my termination take effect?"

"Immediately. Pack up your things. HR will mail you your final paycheck."

Now that surprised me. At least the dean of NJMS had the decency to give me two months' notice. What was even more surprising was that when I got back to my office (right down the hall from his), my phone had already been disconnected and access to my computer had been denied. I borrowed my secretary's phone to call Larry. "I have good news and bad news. The good news is that we can now go on vacation in July. That's because the bad news is I just got my walking papers and I was told to start walking ASAP."

Larry, bless him, took it in stride. He had become a sounding board for the frustration I often expressed after a particularly trying time at work. "It's only 10:00 a.m. What do you plan to do for the rest of the day?" he asked nonchalantly.

"Well, Amas is hosting a special 2:00 p.m. performance of an upcoming musical for people who book group theater tours. It's downtown at the Hudson Guild Theatre where it's scheduled to open in November. I think I'll grab a bite to eat and go see it. It will be comforting to sit alone in the dark and lose myself in a musical without having to make small talk with anyone for two and a half hours. How about I bring home takeout from Ruby Foo's for dinner? I should be home around six-ish"

And my intentions went according to plan, except for the part about being silent and alone. Ruth, my seatmate on the left, was a very personable woman who was also traveling solo. There was no one on her left, so I became her audience. She was from Missouri but she and her husband maintained an apartment in Manhattan so they could come in every few months to satiate their appetite for the Big Apple's cultural offerings, especially live theater. I admitted I was also a theater junkie and told her about my involvement with Amas. It seemed to pique her interest immediately.

"What do you know about investing in a show," she inquired.

"I know it's a very risky proposition. Have you heard the saying, 'You can make a killing in the theater, but you can't make a living?' It's usually the first lesson taught to aspiring producers which is why they seek OPM."

"OPM?"

"Other people's money. And the first lesson investors need to learn is don't put any money into a production that you can't afford to lose."

"Well, my husband and I are thinking of taking the plunge. Our son is a lawyer so we would run everything by him before handing over a check. We came to NYC for the week to see shows in development with the idea of finding one with a minimum level of investment that we could afford. This one sounded promising."

The house lights began to dim, and the overture started up. We sat back to watch *Little Ham*, the nickname of the show's diminutive leading man, Hamilton Hitchcock Jones.

After the show ended to a rousing standing ovation, we turned to each other with big smiles on our faces. "Well, Ruth, I hope you enjoyed it."

"I loved it," she exclaimed. "It's one of the best things I've seen since we've been coming to NY these past few years. I will have to talk it over with my husband, but I think this could be the one we've been waiting for."

"I loved it as well. Here, take my card. If you're serious about investing, I will put you in touch with Eric Krebs, the chairman of the board at Amas and the show's lead producer. Either way, let's keep in contact."

About two weeks later, Ruth called to say that she and her husband had decided to put in $9,000, the minimum needed to become an investor in a hoped-for transfer to a commercial off-Broadway run scheduled to begin at the John Houseman Theater in the fall of 2002.

Up until then I hadn't paid much attention to how theater

productions were financed and didn'; realize that investors could opt in at varying price points. The figure Ruth quoted seemed very doable in light of my NJMS severance package and my anticipated unemployment insurance courtesy of NYCPM. It was then that I decided to make my initial foray into investing. It turned out to be my first encounter with just how fickle the world of commercial theater producing could be. Witness these excerpts from articles before and after the opening at the Houseman:

Kenneth Jones, Playbill, January 6, 2002
Sold-out *Little Ham* Ends Off Broadway January 6… but Dreams of Commercial Hog Heaven

"Still a-tingle from a loving review from *The New York Times*, *Little Ham*, embraced as a crafty, *Guys and Dolls*-style Harlem jazzical, ends its run January 6, with producer Eric Krebs still exploring a commercial future for the piece. The Depression-set musical based on the [Langston] Hughes play of the same name (about the white mob putting pressure on the Harlem numbers racket) is filled with pungent characters typical of the folk who populated works by Hughes, Zora Neale Hurston and other Harlem Renaissance writers."

Michael Portantiere, TheaterMania, September 27, 2002
Producer Eric Krebs Perplexed by Bruce Weber's Re-Review of *Little Ham* for *The New York Times*

"Eric Krebs – lead producer of the musical *Little Ham*, which opened last night at the John Houseman Theater, is 'perplexed' by the fact that Bruce Weber of *The New York Times* wrote a largely negative review of the production after having filed an extremely positive assessment of the show in its previous incarnation at the Hudson Guild Theater late last year. 'It seems to me he is foolishly inconsistent in some ways,' says Krebs of Weber. 'In his first review, he said that the show had a 'high-spirited, melodic score in an indigenous American idiom.' Now he says that 'the score... doesn't exactly feel new. Redolent of the Harlem Renaissance, it owes its main debt to Duke Ellington.' It's the same score played by the same musicians.

'Also, the first time around he wrote that 'in the title role, Andre Garner couldn't be better cast' and he described him as a 'lithe and agile performer.' Now he writes that it 'somehow doesn't add up to a leading man performance.'"

Krebs says there is no question that the show was remounted largely on the basis of Weber's initial notice. "In extremely difficult circumstances, that review made it more possible to raise the money."

In early September 2002, a few weeks before the show's off Broadway opening, I experienced another encounter with synchronicity during a conversation with Bobby, a distant cousin. Bobby told me about an invitation-only career workshop run by a mutual relative named Carole Hyatt. Bobby described Carole as "a pioneering and hyperconnected New Yorker" whose career as an author, motivational speaker, and successful entrepreneur dated back to the early 1960s. Many years later, the sudden death of her business partner in front of her eyes was a paradigm-shifting event in her life. Another contributing factor was her epiphany that the expectation of lifetime employment capped by a gold watch upon retirement needed to be reexamined as technological and social forces began to increasingly reshape the workforce.

The impact was especially hard on women whose career trajectories tended to be less linear than men's, especially if they had taken time out to have and care for children. To empower women, give them coping skills to deal with difficult transitions, and help them reinvent themselves, she had founded the Carole Hyatt Leadership Forum. Its signature event was "Getting to Next," a two-day networking retreat held in her spacious Upper West Side apartment several times throughout the year.

Though I'd never met Carole, Bobby continued to update me about her. I confided in him that I had suffered "the agony of defeet" after getting fired from the podiatry school but didn't feel quite ready to seek the thrill of victory that comes with landing a new job. He offered to contact Carole on my behalf to see if she would consider inviting me to her next workshop. I am generally skeptical of motivational speakers and seminars that, like Uncle Sam, promise to help you "be all that you can be," but I halfheartedly gave him the green light to proceed. A few days later, Carole's assistant called to invite me to the upcoming "Getting to Next" scheduled for Friday and Saturday, September 27 and 28.

Giddy with excitement from hobnobbing with theater luminaries at Chez Josephine for *Little Ham*'s after-party on the evening of Thursday, September 26, I had gone to bed very late that night. I set my alarm for 7:00 a.m. to ensure I would have plenty of time to get to Carole's apartment for the start of the 9:00 a.m. workshop. When my alarm rang, I was tempted to blow off the event altogether in favor of some much needed sleep. But I had paid a hefty amount of (nonrefundable) money to reserve my spot, so I got dressed and got going.

I debated stopping at my corner newsstand to pick up a copy

of *The New York Times* to see if the weekend Arts section contained a review of *Little Ham* but decided against it. I didn't want to risk showing up late to an event where there would be only twenty-five attendees. So I was unaware of Bruce Weber's less than glorious review when I arrived at The Beresford, Carole's prewar, Central Park apartment building opposite the American Museum of Natural History. The uniformed doorman motioned me to the ornate elevator that opened to reveal a uniformed elevator operator waiting to transport me to Carole's floor, which contained only two apartments. The door to the one on the right was ajar so I slipped in and took the one remaining seat in Carole's large, sunny dining room that doubled as The Leadership Forum's conference room.

The agenda began with the customary practice of introductions. However, Carole's instructions for doing them were not customary—at least not to me. She began by stating the goal of her program was to help us discover the core purpose in our lives, and use it as a compass to find a career, volunteer opportunity, or retirement hobby that incorporated it. To get the ball rolling, she told us to envision our dream job or position, and then introduce ourselves as if we already had it.

"Stand up, say your name, and using the past tense, state your current or most recent employment status. Then I want you to use the present tense to tell us what you dream of doing or being as if you are already engaged in it." Her words reminded me of that famous mantra from the Kevin Costner movie, *Field of Dreams*: "If you build it, they will come." In this case, we were being told to envision "it" as if it had already happened.

Her approach threw me for a loop. I had come expecting to sit back and take in whatever inspiring wisdom she was prepared to dispense. Now I had to think fast to come up with my fantasy "next." I didn't have a clue. Luckily, since I was the last person to arrive, I would be the last person called on to introduce myself. I mentally calculated I had about fifteen minutes to come up with something. Still nothing by the time it was my turn at bat. I stood up to speak and uttered the first thought that came to mind.

"Hello. My name is Joan Liman. I used to be a dean of students and admissions at two health professions schools and now I am…a producer." Little did I know that when I uttered those words I would be expected to stick to that vision statement during all of Carole's written and verbal exercises over the next two days. Had I been aware of Weber's unflattering rereview of *Little Ham*, I doubt I would have committed myself to such a precarious profession—even in the low-stakes setting of a career workshop. Nevertheless, there was no going back.

Ever the obedient student, I buckled down and eventually found myself thoroughly immersed in, and actually enjoying, Carole's process. Throughout the day we were split up into breakout groups and dispersed to different rooms in the beautifully decorated apartment to tackle a variety of assignments. (This was real estate hog heaven for me, an inveterate visitor to weekend open houses.) One such task was to articulate our core purpose—the goals that remain constant throughout our lives even if what we do for a living doesn't—then develop a brand name and tagline that embodied it. After considerable brainstorming, I realized caring for people's biopsychosocial needs had been my life's goal and I tried to reflect on this.

The concluding session on Saturday was a lesson in the art of the give and get, aka networking. Each of us was given two minutes to address the group in our new persona, describe our project, clearly state what we needed to get it off the ground, and offer something of value in return. Here's the pitch I gave:

"I am the founder of LimanAde Productions, a nonprofit organization. Our mission is healing hearts through the performing arts. I need donor leads or vendors able to provide in-kind services (e.g., performance venues, sound systems, videography, public relations, etc.) to bring our productions from page to stage. In return, I have an extensive Rolodex and I will be happy to play matchmaker for your professional needs, I am also available to speak to groups or individuals about my personal experience with life-threatening illness. Lastly, I can offer my Sutton Place garden apartment for social or professional gatherings of up to twelve people."

That is how Robb Hunt wound up being my brunch guest five years later. When Robb suggested that I meet Virginia, he was unaware that I had started as a volunteer at Amas and had been asked to take on more responsibility as time went by. He just thought Virginia and I would hit it off because our personalities were so alike. In jest, I joked, "You mean she's an outspoken, native New York Jewish broad like me."

When I reached Virginia, I learned that her parents had settled in a Chicago suburb after fleeing the Nazis but that she was raised as a Methodist. She was practicing family law in Palm Springs, divorced, and remarried with two grown children. As we continued our "getting to know you" chitchat, she mentioned she had commissioned a musical about Hitler's so-called "model city for the Jews," a ghetto/concentration camp located in a former fortress about an hour outside of Prague. A developmental production was currently playing at Robb Hunt's Village Theater. I asked Virginia if she had ever heard of Amas Musical Theatre or its artistic producing director and suggested she submit the script and score to

Donna for consideration as it sounded like it matched the Amas mission.

Her response? "I did but never heard back." To which I blithely replied, "Well, I happen to be the president of the Amas board of directors. Maybe I can help you." So began our journey to bring her musical then titled *Terezin* to New York.

Chapter 31

Signs Of Life

Song: "Hallelujah" sung by Leonard Cohen

Motivated by what I had learned at the "Getting to Next" pro-gram, I began job hunting for what would turn out to be my last paid position. In October 2003, I was hired as the deputy to the medical director and assistant dean of graduate medical educa-tion at Metropolitan Hospital, the facility where I had done my first medical clerkship. By then, Larry was beginning to test the waters of retirement by spending less time at work and more on the golf course. He wanted to take longer and more frequent vacations, but it was difficult to schedule them since I was still holding down a full-time job.

After four-plus years at Metropolitan, I made him a promise: I would retire the year I turned sixty-five or when our first grand-child was due to be born. Ryan entered the world on Tuesday, June 10, 2008, five days after my retirement party. Within a month, the novelty of not having to arise at 6:30 a.m., put on panty hose, don a tailored business suit, and catch the First Avenue bus to go to work every day began to wear off. I started to get restless.

Fortuitously, around the same time I came across a notice in our neighborhood newspaper placed by the Museum of Jewish Heritage—A Living Memorial to the Holocaust seeking volunteers for its Gallery Educator program. "Gall Eds," as they were called, would receive weekly instruction over the course of six months on how to conduct tours of the museum for groups of students as well as community organizations.

The timing was perfect because by then, planning for Virginia's show had already begun ramping up. One of the first producing decisions that had to be made was whether or not to change the show's title. After pitching many ideas, we settled on *Signs of Life*, the name of the title song. The once-a-week docent sessions at the museum gave me a good grounding in WWII history and provided the context for understanding the events that motivated Hitler to create Terezin.

One particular exhibit was exceedingly helpful—a short video narrated by Terezin survivors recalling the time each spent interned in the camp and describing the cunning propaganda scheme devised by the Nazis to dupe an unsuspecting world of the horrors that took place within its fortress walls. A handful were still alive when I began volunteering at the museum, so I was able to meet them in person and recruited several to participate in the post-performance talkbacks regularly scheduled throughout the show's five-week run. One of the most memorable was Fred.

Fred was a tall, lanky fellow with a shock of gray hair whose unassuming demeanor and casual attire made him seem very laid back and unruffled. That image was immediately dispelled when he opened his mouth to talk. He spoke in a very deliberate, even-tempered cadence, choosing his words meticulously and taking dramatic pauses every now and then as if picking the exact phrase was a matter of grave importance.

Fred was in his twenties when he was sent from Prague to Terezin in the early 1940s, where he was assigned to a painting crew in the "beautification effort." After liberation, he settled in the US, studied art, and became a well-known contemporary painter. Some of his work currently hangs in the Smithsonian Institution. When asked why he thought he was able to survive, he paused for a moment, and without a trace of irony, replied, "Good genes and luck." He died in 2022 at the age of ninety-nine.

Another exhibit that left an indelible impression on me was a glass case filled with artifacts, one of which was a pair of well-worn socks donated by Ruth, a fellow Gall Ed. She was the only child of a Polish couple who had owned a very popular confectionary shop. Desperate to save Ruth from being deported, they shared their concerns with one of their customers who then put them in touch with a gentile family willing to take seven-year-old Ruth to live with them in their apartment.

She spent nearly two years as a hidden child, forbidden to go outside and made to hide in a trunk if anyone came to the apartment. She was not allowed to wear shoes when walking around for fear the tenants downstairs might hear her footsteps. Her socks became threadbare and had to be darned over and over to keep them from falling apart. Today, those socks hang in the museum's permanent exhibit, alongside a prewar photo of Ruth as a beautiful, blonde youngster. Ruth included a stop at her socks on every tour she led, waiting until the end to reveal their provenance. By doing so, she helped visitors grasp why the museum had been designed to be a living memorial to the Holocaust. She too is now deceased.

Opening night for *Signs of Life* was scheduled for February 25, 2010. At last, all the time and effort I had expended on this labor of love was about to come to fruition. The prediction of heavy snow beginning in the morning and lasting through late evening couldn't dampen my spirits. I even did some last-minute marketing to the gentleman sitting next to me on the crosstown subway ride to the theater who graciously accepted the flyer I pulled out of my pocketbook. Turns out I had caught the producing bug just as swiftly as I had been infected by the songwriting one back in high school.

Larry was late arriving due to the weather, so I took my seat once the house lights started to dim. I had arranged to sit next to a Terezin survivor who had been introduced to me by Larry's cousin, but I had never met her in person. Anita lived in Westport, Connecticut and volunteered to talk to students throughout the state about her Holocaust experience, which also included stays in Bergen-Belsen, Auschwitz, and a labor camp in Hamburg. During one such school visit, a sixth grader approached her and tentatively asked if he could feel the numbers on her arm. After respectfully brushing his fingers over her tattoo, he reverentially proclaimed, "I've touched history."

At intermission, Anita turned to me with a piercing gaze and clutched my arm. *Uh-oh,* I thought, *she probably hates it and thinks it was blasphemous to make a musical about the terrible place where she was sent when she was only eleven years old.* Instead, with awe in her voice, she said, "Thank you for putting my life on the stage."

At the end of the play, several audience members excitedly asked me, "When is it going to Broadway?" Broadway was also on Larry's mind although he expressed it somewhat differently. With tears in his eyes, he turned to me and said, "Fuck. If this show goes to Broadway, I will never see you!" And though it never made it to the Great White Way, it did have a successful afterlife, thanks in part to Larry's passion and largesse. He was so moved by the show he underwrote a six-week commercial run in Chicago.

Thanks to Gail Humphries, Ph.D., then a professor of theater in the musical theater division at American University (AU), Virginia and I coproduced a number of student readings. Laurie Levy Issembert, a Bethesda, Maryland-based director/producer who had introduced us to Gail, helped mount the first of them on the AU campus. From there Virginia, Gail, and I accompanied the student troupe to Prague, where a reading was performed at the 2013 annual conference of the International Psychoanalytical Association. That year's theme was the use of theater as a healing tool for Holocaust survivors.

Gail had been invited to give the keynote address, so she persuaded the conference organizers to add a one-night performance of *Signs of Life* to the agenda. Prior to that evening, Virginia and I arranged for the students to have a private tour of Terezin. The highlight was a visit to the Attic Theater located in one of the barracks, where inmates had often gathered to watch fellow prisoners perform. Moved by the historical significance of standing on such hallowed ground, the students decided on the spot to do an impromptu rehearsal of one of the songs from *Signs of Life*.

We reprised this hybrid arrangement the following year when the Florida Holocaust Museum in St. Petersburg hosted the annual meeting of the Association of Holocaust Organizations. Yiddishkayt Initiative (YI), a Florida nonprofit organization, had planned on doing a full production in Miami in the spring of 2020 but had to put it on hold due to the arrival of COVID-19. Instead, YI did a virtual reading in April 2021 to commemorate International Holocaust Remembrance Day. It was preceded by a streamed lecture about Terezin delivered by Robert Watson, Ph.D., an award-winning author, professor, historian, and frequent media commentator.

More than twenty years have passed since I stood up in Carole Hyatt's dining room and announced, "I want to be a producer." Since then, I have invested in and helped produce several shows and partnered with Linda Selman, a noted NYC actor, writer, and director to form Me and You Productions to solicit and present work exploring contemporary biopsychosocial issues. I also produced and directed a documentary commemorating the seventy-fifth anniversary of the end of WWII and the liberation of the camps, volunteered and raised funds for YI, and penned three shows of my own: *Cinderella–Not Your Father's Fable*, *A Mensch for Mom*, and *A LimanAde Life: A Little Musical Comedy about Life's Big Tragedies*, upon which this memoir is based.

But none of these have brought me as much *nachas* (proud pleasure) and gratification as *Signs of Life*. It is emblematic of YI's current mission to "battle anti-Semitism through the arts," a vow more crucial than ever in a world that seems to have forgotten an earlier one: "Never again." The bitter truth is, "Never again" is now as evidenced by this February 22, 2023 headline in the *New York Daily News*: "Outrage on Broadway as neo-Nazi group rallies outside *Parade*, a musical about a lynched American Jew."

The show is based on the true story of Leo Frank. Frank was accused and convicted of the 1913 rape and murder of a teenage girl working at the Georgia factory where he was employed as the superintendent. The Anti-Defamation League (ADL) was founded in the wake of the Leo Frank case with the short-term goal of stopping defamation of the Jewish people. The ultimate goal, according to its 1913 charter, was "to secure justice and fair treatment to all citizens alike and to put an end forever to unjust and unfair discrimination against and ridicule of any sect or body of citizens."

Sadly, more than a century has passed since that mission statement was put forth and yet that goal still seems elusive. The past decade has seen a steady erosion of the democratic rights that most Americans had complacently come to consider the norm. The political progress embodied in the civil rights movement of the 1960s that legalized the voting rights of blacks is being undermined by state efforts such as redlining and gerrymandering; likewise, overturning the landmark 1973 Supreme Court case of Roe vs. Wade in June 2022 unleashed a spate of harsh antiabortion laws, some of which criminalize the termination of a pregnancy even in circumstances where the life of the woman is in danger.

In 1994, then senator, Joe Biden worked hard to pass an Assault Weapons Ban that had a ten-year sunset provision. After Republicans allowed it to expire in 2004, mass shootings tripled to the point where according to data released by the Gun Violence Archive, one hundred mass shootings had occurred between January 1 and March 7, 2023, an average of one shooting a day.

Police brutality is another recurring problem, made more visible in recent years thanks to body cams worn by officers and amateur video recordings taken by nearby bystanders, as was made brutally apparent in the murders of Breonna Taylor, George Floyd, and Tyre Nichols. And I never would have imagined that I would wind up spending my retirement years in a state where book banning has come to be considered sound educational practice. Elected officials in Florida are censoring black history by legislating it out of its schools and "Don't Say Gay" has become the de facto state motto.

As my license plate proclaims, I live in the Sunshine State, but storm clouds began hovering over it around the 2018 midterm elections, just about the same time I became a permanent resident. I felt like I was experiencing a year-round case of SAD (Seasonal

Affective Disorder), an apt acronym for what I was feeling. When the 2020 arrival of the pandemic prompted a lockdown, my malaise ramped up. To preserve my sanity—and keep me from gaining the COVID-19—I began churning out song parodies with a decidedly partisan slant and enlisted a creative team to turn them into YouTube music videos a la my idol, Randy Rainbow.

While they garnered praise and generated some followers, I felt an obligation to take a more proactive stance as the 2020 election cycle started heating up. Heeding the words of Martin Luther King, Jr.—"Our lives begin to end the day we become silent about things that matter"—I held and attended fundraisers, donated money, participated in pro-choice marches, mailed postcards, and made phone calls in support of Democratic candidates running at all governmental levels.

In addition to my advocacy work with the 451 Avengers, I combined my passion for musical theater with my outrage against injustice by joining the South Florida chapter of Raging Grannies. It is an international group of older female activists who write and perform song parodies in parks, at rallies, in front of governmental buildings, and even on street corners to heighten awareness of and protest societal wrongs.

And in the wake of the Israel-Hamas war I signed petitions, attended vigils, posted numerous Facebook messages with my signature affixed to them, and proudly displayed an Israeli flag on my doorstep, and a Jewish star around my neck while simultaneously expressing concern for the humanitarian crisis unfolding in Gaza.

On February 23, 2024, I turned seventy-five. Looking back, I would like to think that I lived a life in accordance with the Jewish precept of *tikkun olam*—Hebrew for repairing the world. This idea also resonates with the inscription engraved on the headstone of boxing legend and humanitarian Muhammad Ali, one of the most celebrated American converts to Islam. It reads: *Service to others is the rent you pay for your room in heaven.*

I hope that my rent will have been paid in full by the time I am laid to rest.

Epilogue

I'm Still Standing

Song: "I'm Still Standing" sung by Elton John

Hot, cloudy with a 35 percent chance of late afternoon thunderstorms.

That was the morning forecast for May 22, 2021 – the day of my grandson Ryan's bar mitzvah in New Jersey where fairly strict COVID-19 regulations were still in place. Although the synagogue had recently begun to allow on-site services (albeit with restricted attendance), the reception was to be held outside at a nearby restaurant under a protective roof-like structure installed over part of the parking lot. There were no side flaps, so guests would not be entirely sheltered from heavy rain or strong gusts of wind.

Nevertheless, my spirits refused to be dampened as I drove to the hair salon at 7:30 a.m. to get beautified. Thanks to the magic hands of the stylist and makeup artist, I was transformed from my every day, unadorned self into a "glam-ma." And with the help of two layers of Spanx undergarments and a pair of "chicken cutlets" (the fashion-industry's term for uplifting adhesive breast pads with poultry-like consistency that eliminated the need to wear a bra under my formfitting, off-the-shoulder, tomato red Badgley Mischka dress bought on sale), I morphed into full-on dazzling diva. The coup de grace was the panoply of diamond jewelry my husband had given me over the course of fifty-five years of marriage, most of which rarely saw the light of day because it was sequestered in a bank vault except for special occasions.

From the moment Larry and I pulled up to Temple Beth Tik-vah, it was apparent a pandemic-style event would be taking place. Only a handful of cars were visible, looking forlorn in a parking lot that would ordinarily be filled to overflowing for a Saturday morning bar or bat mitzvah in a reform congregation. As we crossed the threshold, the first person we encountered was a female police officer sporting a bulletproof black vest and matching mask. She was guarding a table holding personalized yarmulkes embroidered with my grandson's name and the words *Cleared for takeoff*.

They nestled alongside custom-made masks made out of the same material, sporting the initial of his first name in a jaunty, bold-faced font. I doubted the guest list included any anti-maskers but just in case, the officer's handgun was visibly displayed in her holster should enforcement become necessary.

Entering the sanctuary felt eerily like stepping into a religious ghost town. Built to accommodate five hundred worshipers, only twenty-five souls were permitted to occupy it that morning. Melanie is an only child and my immunocompromised, childless sister lived in Florida where the pandemic kept her confined to her home, so most of them were guests of Melanie's former husband. Besides his new wife, they included my former *machatunim*—his parents (or as I fondly call them "macha-tuna fish"), his two sisters and their plus-ones, some of his aunts and uncles, and their respective offspring.

The passage of time since my daughter's divorce enabled all of us to gather cordially and exchange sincere pleasantries; if not for social-distancing protocol, we would have probably exchanged hugs and kisses as well. I offered my heartfelt congratulations to my former son-in-law and told his wife my grandchildren were very fortunate to have her in their lives because she was such a caring and devoted stepmother. She'd even learned some Hebrew so she could stand on the bimah and recite the prayer customarily offered before reading a section of the Torah. As the two female officiants, Rabbi Meeka and Cantor Erica, entered the sanctuary signaling the start of the service, I offered my own prayer to acknowledge how grateful I was that things had turned out well for all parties concerned.

The rabbi and the cantor stood on opposite ends of the bimah, each protected by a plastic shield as if they were museum artifacts, further contributing to the artifice of the setting. Equidistant between them was my grandson, positioned behind a lectern nearly his height. He barely cleared five feet, so this was to be expected. It was the first time I had ever seen him in a suit, and he looked so handsome.

What did surprise me was that a Torah scroll lay unfurled on the lectern before the service had even begun. Normally it remains behind the closed doors of the arc until it is time to read the week's portion. The scroll gets handed from grandparent to parent to child to symbolize the passing of the laws of God from one generation to the next (l'dor va dor). Apparently, this was another part of collateral damage to religious life in the age of the Corona virus. The hands-on ritual that is such a treasured moment in the ceremony had been mandated to become hands-off.

As I tried to wrap my head around all of this, I found my

thoughts wandering back to my daughter's bat mitzvah—October 5, 1985. Rather than the glorious fall weather I had hoped for, the morning dawned overcast and chilly. But nothing was going to dampen my spirits that day since I never thought I would get to live long enough to see it. After all, I had defied the odds and outlived my expiration date several times over.

My father had passed away the previous January so he wouldn't get to participate in one of the most significant milestones in the life of his only grandchild. But my mother was still very much alive as evidenced by the heavy tread of her steps in our upstairs bedroom where she had been installed after her arrival a few days earlier. She had flown up from Florida for the occasion and, much to the chagrin of my husband, would be staying for a week. (Apparently, she had never heard the adage about houseguests and three-day-old fish.)

The guest list had included forty or so of Melanie's nearest and dearest friends, so I'd made arrangements for several carpools to transport them from Temple Beth Or to the nearby hotel that had been booked for the reception immediately following the service. After downing a hasty breakfast, my husband and Melanie set out for the synagogue in his car as she had to be there thirty minutes before the designated 10:00 a.m. start time. Old habits dying hard, my mother was still upstairs in her room getting dressed because she had never mastered the time management skills required to arrive somewhere on time. After several pleas to hurry up, we finally made it out the door and into the garage. More precious minutes passed while she made several fumbled attempts to put on her seat belt. Finally, in a fit of desperation, I impatiently reached across her ample chest, grabbed the buckle from her hand, shoved it into its receptacle, slammed my foot on the gas pedal, and backed out of the garage, nearly shearing off my side mirror in the process.

We entered the sanctuary just as Rabbi Berkowitz announced, "We will begin the service on page 175 of your prayer books." I beamed with pride as he called upon Melanie to recite the first of the many passages she would read throughout the morning. My smile grew even brighter when the Torah scroll was removed from the arc and the rabbi asked Larry and me to come stand next to her to chant the customary blessings said before reading from that week's *parshah* or section. When we ascended the three steps to the bimah, however, I suddenly felt my eyes welling up with tears as I recalled that fateful June day in my hospital room some four years earlier when I was told I probably wouldn't live until my thirty-fourth birthday, yet here I was celebrating her thirteenth. Silently, I offered my thanks to God for what truly seemed to be a miracle.

Shortly afterward, a strange thing happened. Mere minutes into my daughter's recitation of her Torah portion, there was a bolt of lightning, a loud clap of thunder, and finally, the sound of torrential rain reverberating throughout the sanctuary. Within seconds, the roof over the bimah began leaking sending people in the first few pews scuttling to higher ground behind them. To my daughter's credit, she remained unfazed and continued to chant along to what I was sure was God's accompaniment to celebrate my presence on an important milestone in my only child's life.

After saying the traditional blessings over the bread and wine, I assigned Melanie's friends to the various vehicles that would take them to the hotel where the reception was slated to start at one pm. Our family car at the time was a Chevy station wagon that could accommodate seven people, including my mother and me. Since it was still raining heavily, I told her to wait under the overhang of the synagogue's front door and I would swing by to pick her up so she wouldn't have to traipse out to the parking lot. Once I managed to get five adolescents to stop fighting about who would get to sit in the "way back," I took off for the hotel. It wasn't until the franks in blankets had finished being passed around that I realized I had left my mother behind. Just as I was about to dash off and retrieve her, she magically appeared.

Luckily, the sisterhood president had been in attendance at the service to present Melanie with the gifts customarily bestowed on the boy or girl entering adulthood—a Kiddush cup and prayer book. As she exited, she saw my mother forlornly huddled under an umbrella and offered to give her a lift. Once my heart stopped pounding, I embraced my mom and started to apologize profusely. I didn't get very far before she spotted relatives she hadn't seen in forever and left me to embrace them. Once again, I felt that God was in my corner because the distraction literally rescued me from what could have been a very tight spot.

My reverie was cut short by the sound of Rabbi Meeka strumming her guitar to signal Ryan's bar mitzvah was about to begin. She called his parents up to the bimah where his father placed a tallis, a ceremonial shawl, around his shoulders, signifying his entrance into manhood. The service started out with the *Shehecheyanu*, a traditional prayer recited at the start of most Jewish holidays as well as one that celebrates the first time something occurs.

The self-assurance and composure with which Ryan led the congregants in reciting these words, never once faltering in his delivery, belied the recalcitrance and resistance he had exhibited in preparing for his rite of passage. This stubborn streak grew even stronger when he started attending the bar mitzvahs of his friends, many of whom had birthdays that preceded his. Adam Stein was one of them.

Adam attended Beth El, a synagogue that was even less traditional than Beth Torah. Much of the service there was conducted in English, so the students in its b'nai mitzvah classes didn't have to master as much material and had smaller roles in leading it. Up until Adam's bar mitzvah, Ryan had never attended any other synagogue than his own, so this was an eye-opener for him. Unbeknownst to his parents, Ryan texted Rabbi Meeka and Cantor Erica to express his annoyance at this seeming injustice. He proclaimed how unfair it was that he had to learn so much more than Adam and told them he ought to be allowed to "downsize" his participation.

Naturally, Ryan and his parents were summoned to meet with both women. They patiently explained to him that rituals differ from synagogue to synagogue and that almost all the Hebrew school students they had shepherded throughout their combined years of service had become increasingly more nervous as their assigned dates grew closer. Rabbi Meeka even confided that her own daughter had given her a hard time. Ryan ultimately shared that he had never liked being the center of attention in social situations and was uncomfortable at the thought that so many eyes would be focused on him during the two-hour service.

Despite his long-standing reluctance to stand in the spotlight, he had been able to make his presence known by the small acts of kindness he'd exhibited from an early age. On a trip to Dollywood during Ryan's early elementary school years, Larry and I had taken him to the gift shop one morning while Marissa was still sleeping. When we told him he could pick out anything he wanted, his first response was, "What about Marissa? We have to get something for her." Only after we reassured Ryan we would take care of that, he went off to select his own present. We were taken aback when he showed up at the cash register with a "grabber"—the ingenious device that is used to retrieve items that are hard to reach. In retrospect, the practicality of that purchase foreshadowed his penchant for problem solving and logistics.

After he attended his middle school orientation, he came home and plotted out the respective routes he and his best friend would be using to navigate the school's corridors during change of classes and plotted where their paths might cross along the way. As he got older, we relied on him to be our GPS guide during road trips. If our travel plans including flying, he would be the one to determine what time we should leave to get to the airport, then calculate our itinerary with the military precision befitting a four-star general, indicating our ETAs at the intermediate points along the route. For the twenty-seven-mile drive from our Florida home to West Palm Beach to catch a 4:00 p.m. flight boarding at 2:15 p.m., his schedule looked like this:

12:55 p.m. - leave the house

12:57 p.m. - exit the gates of our condo community

1:10 p.m. - arrive at on-ramp for I-95

1:35 p.m. - get off at Exit 69 (Belvedere Road)

1:38 p.m. - enter airport parking lot

1: 43 p.m. - walk to JetBlue terminal

1:50 p.m. - check in and go through security

2:15 p.m. - walk to gate for departure to Newark

2: 20 p.m. - arrive at gate

3:15 p.m. - await call to board

Ryan's thoughtfulness manifested itself outside the immediate family. One of Melanie's close friends had a child about the same age as Ryan. Tyler was on the spectrum and attended a special needs school. Their mothers arranged play dates for them and Tyler really took to him because of his kindhearted nature. Ryan was just as thoughtful to his own classmates, which earned him two awards from his teachers attesting to his willingness to help others. To quote Edith Wharton, "There are two ways of spreading light: to be the candle or the mirror that reflects it." Ryan shone when it came to helping other people shine.

Once Ryan's bar mitzvah apprehension was out in the open, the rabbi and cantor pledged to work with him in the remaining weeks to make the experience as comfortable as possible. His parents still had some apprehension about if he would be able to pull it off.

When he confidently strode to the lectern and began reading from the prayer book in a calm, controlled manner, my daughter and I exchanged looks of amazement. Was this the same individual who had refused to pose or smile for the professional photographer she had hired to take pictures the night before? You'd never know it from the self-assured teenager who stood before us, a poster boy for poise under pressure. On that day he was the candle.

Even the rabbi and cantor were pleasantly surprised. During their congratulatory remarks, they acknowledged that coaching Ryan over the past few months had proved to be quite a challenge and how proud they were of his performance. The cantor went one step further by declaring that Ryan's stubborn streak could prove to be a positive attribute going forward if he applied it to a constructive purpose whether it be persevering in the face of obstacles to achieve his personal best in a competitive sport or supporting a worthy but perhaps unpopular cause.

By the time it was my granddaughter's turn to ascend the bimah on the day of her bat mitzvah, social-distancing restrictions were no longer in place and masks were optional. The guest list had expanded to one hundred and forty, including fifty-three of her friends. Unlike her brother, Marissa enjoyed being in the spotlight. From the time she was a preschooler, one of her favorite activities when her grandfather and I came to visit was "putting on a show." She would usher us to the living room couch while she went "backstage" (i.e., the hallway) to prepare for her entrance.

She cast me as the emcee, and I was more than happy to oblige. "Ladies and gentlemen, presenting the one, the only, the great Marissa." Then she would break into song and pantomime the gestures of whatever teenage pop star was at the top of the charts.

She was also very good at impersonations. Her best was a spot-on impression of Veruca Salt, the wealthy, spoiled brat in *Willy Wonka and the Chocolate Factory* who petulantly whines her way through the song, "I Want it Now," in a high British accent. She did a pretty good Australian one too. When TikTok arrived on the scene, Marissa became an ardent devotee. Her videos featured her singing songs or acting out original scenarios complete with props and costumes. Often, she would recruit me to make a cameo appearance. She proved to be a demanding director. "No, Nonny, you made your entrance too soon. Go back and do it again." Her burgeoning comic skills were also put to good use in the creation of these skits. In fifth grade, her teacher told my daughter that Marissa was the funniest student in the class.

I'd like to think that she inherited her comedic DNA from me. I had always prided myself on having a good sense of humor and being able to able to find something to chuckle about, even in situations that didn't seem to warrant laughter. It's like that old Jewish riddle: "What is the definition of a Jewish holiday? 'They tried to kill us, we survived, let's eat.'" My inspiration was sparked by Norman Lear, the iconic television writer and producer described in a 2023 *New York Times* article as "being responsible for bringing a fuller picture of Black lives to American TV screens." Marla Gibbs, who rose to fame as Florence, the maid in *The Jeffersons,* remembers him telling her shortly before his death at 101 that "laughter adds years to one's life."

When I began to manifest some of the side effects of my lymphoma treatment regimen in the summer of 1981, I joked, "Let me tell you about the new wonder diet I'm on: it makes you lose weight…and hair." And when I learned that Dr. Dopa Mean specialized in psychiatry, I quipped, "Giving it, not treating it," a punch line that always got a chortle from my colleagues.

Even at the tender age of two, Ryan appreciated my talent. He was squirming on the diaper changing table while I was trying to clean him up. To distract him, I started to make funny faces and blew a raspberry on his tummy. He stopped, smiled up at me and said, "Nonny, you make me laugh."

Marissa was also somewhat of a drama queen, and her wit could be tinged with sarcasm. The summer before she started fourth grade, we were swimming in the pool at my NJ retirement community when a neighbor, a former schoolteacher, paddled over to say hello.

"Marissa, this is my good friend Lydia."

Marissa was too busy noodling with her pool noodle to acknowledge the introduction. Lydia graciously filled the void.

"It's very nice to meet you, Marissa. I've heard a lot about you. You just finished third grade, right?"

My granddaughter made a grunt of acknowledgement and

went back to playing with the pool toy. In an effort to elicit a more polite reply, I put my hand on the noodle and gave her a stern look. In my best "here's a fun fact" voice, I said, "Lydia used to teach third grade." To which Marissa dismissively retorted, "Good for her."

As she got older, Marissa would reprimand me if she didn't approve of something I said or did. "Nonny, you're embarrassing me" or "That's so rude, Nonny" were two of her favorite rebukes. But she could also melt my heart at the most unexpected times. During a pre-COVID-19 winter vacation, Melanie brought her and Ryan to visit Larry, aka Pop Pop, and me in Florida. They were booked on a late afternoon flight back to NJ on New Year's Day so we went to brunch in our club's main dining room around 10:00 a.m. Marissa chose to order an omelet while Ryan opted to go to the elaborate buffet. She had already started eating when he came back with a stack of pancakes. She frowned and said she wanted pancakes too. When I refused to acquiesce, the frown turned into a full-on pout, but I remained steadfast. As a concession, I promised to make her pancakes for lunch, and she settled down.

Later, as she was rolling her suitcase down our driveway toward the airport-bound Uber idling at the curb, she stopped, threw her arms around my waist, hugged me tightly, and gave me an unsolicited compliment. "Nonny, you're terrific. I'm gonna miss you a lot."

When it came time to prepare for her bat mitzvah, I felt sure Marissa's moxie would stand her in good stead and she wouldn't hang back as her brother had. I was so convinced that while I was browsing the card rack of a local Hallmark store well in advance of her birthday, I decided on the spot to buy a card that seemed custom-made for her. It read, "A Sassy, Classy, Badassy Lassie from

NJ–Nobody does you like you do. Happy birthday." Imagine my surprise when my daughter informed me that Marissa was balking at putting in the necessary effort to master the Torah portion and prayers she was required to perform.

Like most teenagers her age, she spent her spare time wedded to her cell phone. Prying it out of her hand and putting it out of her reach to get her to sit down and study was a Herculean effort. In a repeat performance from 2021, about two months before her bat mitzvah date, Marissa's parents were once again asked to meet with the current rabbi and cantor (their predecessors had left to take other positions soon after Ryan's bar mitzvah). Both officiants opined that Marissa wouldn't be ready if she didn't improve her efforts.

By the time I heard the news, only three weeks remained for her to catch up. I told my daughter I was willing to meet with Marissa once a week to put her through her paces and wouldn't put up with any stonewalling on her part. Lo and behold, just like her brother, she rose to the occasion Marissa took command of the lectern with the self-assurance and posture of a celebrity. She even resembled one in her ruffled white organza dress with rhinestone-studded belt and matching barrette. It appeared as if she was to the pulpit born. After she was done, the rabbi draped his arm around her shoulders and said, "That was amazing." With her characteristic aplomb, she gave a nonchalant shrug and replied, "I know."

He also drew attention to her altruism when he told the congregation how Marissa had fulfilled the synagogue's community service requirement. Of the various options available, she chose to volunteer at a local senior citizens' center where she took part in various recreation activities with its residents. In recognition of her efforts, she was chosen to give a speech at a ceremony honoring volunteers. He concluded by announcing that in the aftermath of the October 7, 2023 Hamas terrorist attacks on Israel, Marissa had offered to donate a portion of her bat mitzvah gift money to Israel.

At that moment, I realized the tenacity and perseverance of both my grandchildren would enable them to adhere to one of the most fundamental precepts of Judaism regardless of their future levels of observance—*tikkun olam*—to repair the world; to make it a little better place than it was before you entered it. Given the current state of global affairs, this will not be an easy task for their generation, but they have already demonstrated they will be up to the challenge.

I also had another epiphany: Ryan and Marissa weren't the only ones in our family with a stubborn streak. After all, if not for my relentless resiliency in the face of multiple hardships, I probably would not have lived to see them transform into adults right before my eyes. I knew the *Shehecheyanu* in Hebrew by rote and, up until then, had paid only cursory attention to its English translation. After the privilege of witnessing their coming-of-age, I realized that I was the living embodiment of its message:

"Blessed are You, Lord our God, Ruler of the Universe, who has given us life, sustained us, and allowed us to reach this day."

Finale

Song: "A LimanAde Life" Music and Lyrics by Joan Liman

If I hadn't gotten married
At the age of twenty-one
An age that's now considered
To be really rather young
Would I have developed into
Who I have become?
Well, I'll never know.

If I'd moved to New York City
When my college years were through
Shared a fifth-floor walk up
That was meant for one not two
Would I have a penthouse now
Three bedrooms, river view?
Well, I'll never know.

Were life a cosmic chess game

We'd live strategically
Each move we'd make,
Each step we'd take
With calculated glee.

Instead, it's more like poker
You play the hand you're dealt
Sometimes you hit the jackpot
Or you're hit below the belt.

If I hadn't had a mother
Needing mothering herself
Whose stash of tranquilizers
Took up one entire shelf
Would I now have a cleaner bill
Of so-called "mental health"
Kinda hard to tell.

If the ravages of illness
Hadn't left their mark on me
And I'd completed training
In my chosen specialty
Might I have found the
Wonder drug for curing HIV?
Wouldn't have that been swell!

But life is like a highway
From cradle to the grave
For some it's just a straight road
On blacktop primly paved

In my case, bumpy back roads
Some quite circuitous
Were my main mode of travel
But they still led to success.

If I were asked the question
"Would you change a thing or two?"
In retrospect I'd have to say
(spoken)
Who wouldn't, wouldn't you?

But squeezing all my lemons
Into Liman lemonade
Resulted in a frothy brew
That I'm now serving up to you

And with it, here's a tidbit
A slice of good advice
It might just come in handy
Once or even twice
If one day you wake up
And the sky is falling down
Try eating clouds for breakfast
They could turn your life around.

Joan Liman, MD

Acknowledgments

"I Could Write a Book," sung by Gene Kelly in the Rodgers and Hammerstein musical, **Pal Joey**

And so, I did. But when I sat down to write this section, I was confronted by a blank page and an acute case of writer's block. Though I had managed to pen more than 60,000 words for a memoir, I was stymied by the prospect of writing a few short, pithy paragraphs acknowledging the individuals from all walks of life who inspired and helped me embark on the literary journey that resulted in *My LimanAde Life.*

And then it dawned on me: I had already done so by virtue of including many of them as characters in the book because they were central to my story. Without their ongoing support, encouragement (and in some cases, well-meaning meddling), I might not have lived long enough to share my "LimanAde" life with you, the reader.

That said, there are still several people who deserve special recognition because they constitute the "supporting cast" that enabled me to bring the book to fruition.

Madeline Mishel Hauptman, my lifelong friend, confidante, and accomplished artist who created a personalized oil painting for me as a get-well gift following my mastectomy. Even though we no longer live near enough to visit each other, I think of her every day when I walk past it as it is prominently displayed in the front entrance hall of my home.

Joan Robbins Foley, my high school classmate and later, college roommate, who introduced me to "Sing," the extracurricular activity that was a turning point in my life and whose poetry attests to her literary talents.

Deborah Tannenbaum, our quirky senior AP English teacher, who instilled our shared love of writing. Her mantra, "Document, document, document," was one of many cautionary admonishments she doled out to emphasize the importance of substantiating the theses we put forth in our papers with examples from the assigned texts. And when I was chosen as one of three commencement speakers, she allowed me to deliver an address filled with humorous anecdotes rather than the usual feel-good bromides, thereby getting the most applause. (I admit it; I'm a ham at heart.)

Lois and Andy Pink plus Wendy and Frank Post and their respective families with whom my husband, daughter, and I shared multiple tumbles, countless cups of hot chocolate, and much laughter during our ski trips out west and whose loyalty and compassion never wavered despite the demands my illnesses made on our friendship over the past half a century.

Loni Figura, MD, is one of the dearest individuals in my life since meeting her during my very first weeks at New York Medical College. The most energetic, vibrant, and game-for-anything woman I have ever met. Despite juggling the demands of motherhood and medicine, she always found time to visit me in my hospital or mental health facility 'de jour,' bring me whimsical gifts, and ply me with homemade gourmet treats in between traveling to Nashville to take a course in writing country music, ski monster moguls in sub-zero temperatures in Utah, and participate in Iron Man Triathlons as far away as California.

Joyia Bradley, writer, director, performer (and dog trainer). Her amazing one-woman play, *Soul To Keep* was my first real producing credit some twenty years ago. Working with her was such a 'joy' that I asked her to direct my fractured fairy tale musical, *Cindercellar: Not Your Father's Fable*. Bob Ost, founder of Theater Resources Unlimited (TRU), who worked with me to get Joyia's show up and running in the Midtown International Theatre Festival and directed as well as wrote music for the earliest incarnations of my show, *A LimanAde Life*. I was delighted to accept his subsequent offer of TRU board membership and honored to be invited to his wedding to his long-time collaborator and partner, Gary Hughes.

Through TRU I met Linda Selman, a highly accomplished actor, director, dramaturge, and author. She taught me the fundamentals of playwriting and reworked my first show into a tighter, more theatrical piece. We took our working relationship to the next level by forming Me and You Productions, a company devoted to presenting plays with contemporary biopsychosocial themes such as Hal Ackerman's *Testosterone: How Prostate Cancer Made a Man Out of Me*. I look forward to our continuing collaboration.

Frank Dagostino, with his good looks, perennial tan, and dapper wardrobe, is the closest I have ever come to knowing a bon vivant. As his Facebook photos attest, he regularly hobnobs with Palm Beach socialites and New York City celebrities, allowing me to live vicariously in both realms. He had a glamourous life as a professional ice skater before performing the musical theater equivalent of a triple axel by spinning his own music, lyrics, and book into a unique Broadway-style show titled *Ice*. Frank's career trajectory gave me the confidence that I too might be able to "go for the gold" and he has become one of my biggest supporters.

Lea Wolinetz, a spunky go-getter and the only person I know who speaks faster than I do. A real plus since she has a plethora of knowledge to convey. The daughter of Holocaust survivors, she has played an active role in commemorating her parents through her dedicated involvement in worldwide "never forget" programs. She was the first person I thought of when asked to recruit new members to the board of Yiddishkayt Initiative. I will be forever grateful that she accepted my offer and for her untiring outreach efforts on behalf of the organization.

I met the late Barbara Sickmen as a result of an acquaintance's casual, last-minute invitation to join her and a few of her companions for a pre-curtain happy hour. Though short in stature, she had a larger-than-life presence and was a born raconteur with prodigious musical talent to boot. Like Frank, Barbara was a theatrical multi-hyphenate. When she discovered I was an aspiring lyricist she took me under her wing to mentor me in the art of songwriting, a random act of kindness that proved to be the start of a beautiful friendship. During our sessions, I'd invariably utter something that appeared to strike a metaphorical chord with her; without warning, she'd spontaneously start to sing one of her own compositions– ostensibly to illustrate a point, one I was often hard-pressed to discern. Or she would eagerly start telling me an anecdote, forgetting she had already relayed it to me many times over. Oh, how I miss her—lovely, loveable, loquacious Barbara.

And merci beaucoup to my editor extraordinaire, Cheryl Benton—the 'coolest' hot tomato I know. Were it not for her involvement from the beginning some five years ago, you would not be holding this volume in your hands. I originally envisioned it as a legacy to my grandchildren containing source material about the life I'd led before becoming their "Nonny." About one-third of the way through the first draft, Cheryl began lobbying me to publish it through her company so it could be marketed to the general public.

Because so much of the content was very personal, I was uneasy about sharing it with readers outside my immediate family. As flattered as I was by her suggestion, I turned her down. Cheryl continued to cajole, and I continued to demur, knowing I would be revealing even more sensitive details in the chapters still to come. When I finally confided this, her reaction convinced me to change my mind. "All the more reason you should publish it. Your candor coupled with your humor will resonate with anyone who has ever been caught up in life-challenging circumstances as well as the loved ones who cheered them on from the sidelines." So, Cheryl, if your prediction happens to come true, feel free to say, "I told you so."

About the Author

Joan Liman, MD, MPH

Joan Liman's passion for theater ignited during Brooklyn's James Madison High School's annual musical, SING. With a BA in Psychology from the State University of NY at Buffalo (Phi Beta Kappa), she pursued medicine at New York Medical College earning her medical degree with honors, along with a master's in public health. Her career spanned roles as associate dean for student affairs at New Jersey Medical School and deputy to the medical director at NYC's Metropolitan Hospital Center.

Upon retiring, Joan decided to "heal hearts through the performing arts," and embraced her lifelong dream: producing and writing for theater. Her off-Broadway producing debut *Signs of Life*, a WWII musical drama, marked the beginning of her creative journey. An award-winning playwright, she champions Yiddishkayt Initiative's battle against antisemitism through the arts. Her favorite roles? Wife, mom, "Nonny," and devoted dog parent. Visit her YouTube page, LimanAde Productions. https://www.youtube.com/@limanadeproductions3050

The proceeds from her book will go to various charities she supports.

www.ingramcontent.com/pod-product-compliance
Lightning Source LLC
Chambersburg PA
CBHW060923120626
46557CB00003B/850